It's All In Your Head
(Diseases Caused By Silver-Mercury Fillings)

For Questions on Recommendations
or Proper Procedures to Follow
Call (800) 331-2303
Monday - Friday, 8 A.M. - 5 P.M.
Mountain Time Zone, U.S.A.

HUGGINS VITAE

Hal A. Huggins, DDS graduated from the University of Nebraska School of Dentistry. He practiced general dentistry with an emphasis on nutrition for over 20 years. For the last eleven years of his practice he tried unsuccessfully to bring to the attention of the dental community the facts he had learned regarding the potential harm patients suffer from dental amalgam fillings. Finally, in 1983 he decided to devote full time to diagnosing and planning treatment for patients with mercury toxicity.

He now spends his days in consultations with patients, either in the office or by phone. When he is not actively involved with patients he is studying at the University of Colorado in the field of immunology in an attempt to provide answers to questions of how mercury affects the immune system. He also spends hours in the development of treatment aids such as supplement formulations to encourage excretion of mercury.

BOOK DESCRIPTION

"Mercury toxicity may well prove to be the most invasive disease of our time" state the Huggins' about this condition afflicting at least 20% of the population of this country.

The method of treatment planning that the Huggins' employ in helping their patients recover from the devastating affects of mercury toxicity is controversial in medical and dental circles at this time. But their success rate is over 80% in terms of reversing symptoms and improving quality of life.

This book will explain in detail---------
> why dental fillings are the primary source of mercury toxicity
> what other sources of mercury can create problems
> what dental materials should be used
> how nutrition affects recovery from mercury toxicity.

It also provides references from dental and medical literature as well as Dr. Huggins' complete presentation to the National Institute of Dental Research Workshop on the Biocompatibility of Dental Materials in July, 1984. These have been added to the book to satisfy questions from professionals, but are made easy to understand by the public as well.

This book can change your life if you are one of the millions of persons suffering from sensitivities to the dental materials in your mouth.

ISBN 0-943685-06-0

Life Sciences Press

DEDICATION

We dedicate this book first to the patients who have suffered needlessly from having mercury in their mouths and secondly to the media who has helped us take this message to those who need to hear it.

We especially thank Tom Bearden of Channel 7 News in Denver, Colorado for his tireless efforts in presenting the entire story and for his concern for the patients whose lives he has touched.

HAT'S OFF
(OTHERWISE KNOWN AS ACKNOWLEDGEMENTS)

"It's best to laugh at your problems if you want to live through them" is the statement portrayed by Chester Commodore's cartoons and his personal life. We feel fortunate to have met this happy illustrator who spent more than twelve hours a day from 1948 forward doing illustrations for The Chicago Defender. As the years went by, he became one of the top political cartoonists in the country. For twelve consecutive years (1968 to 1980) he saw his political cartoons nominated for the Pulitzer Prize. Commodore has the unique ability to capture our ideas and make them live on paper. Our gratitude to you, Commodore.

Our thanks also to the pen and sharp eye of Marcia Kuharich. She began with an objective outsider's view of the subject — her only involvement was to make certain that we said things clearly and correctly. But she finished her editing responsibilities knowing that she, too, is a victim of mercury toxicity. Marcia helped tremendously in showing us how to present exactly what we wanted to say in just the best way. Thanks, Marcia, for your encouragement and help.

TABLE OF CONTENTS

"It is a well known fact that amalgam of every known composition corrodes."
> — Schoonover & Souder, 1941; Mateer and Reitz, 1970

"When mercury is combined with the metals used in dental amalgam, its toxic properties are made harmless."
> — American Dental Association, 1984

PREFACE TO THE THIRD EDITION
by
Hal A. Huggins, D.D.S.

"A lot has happened since I saw you last." This has been a password of people who have been active in the mercury toxicity issue. It has certainly been true in my case. Each month has brought about new ideas, new challenges, new successes, fewer defeats, and a realization of how our society is really structured.

Four years after *All In Your Head* first surfaced, it is time to give an update to new features that answer old questions and show the new year's models of advances in treatment. The 1985 concepts have not changed. Mercury is still bad. It's just that now we know how bad. Diet is still important. It's just that now we know how important. Some day it will be time for a new book. But not today. The war isn't over yet.

Here are some updates on events bringing us to the new decade. Here's to a decade free from a major environmental hazard that is — *All in Your Head.*

ICBM DECLARATION

The International Conference on the Biocompatibility of Materials

declares that:

"Based on the known toxic potentials of mercury and its documented release from dental amalgams, usage of mercury-containing amalgam increases the health risk of the patients, the dentists, and dental personnel."

The above statement is a landmark conclusion for dentistry. It demonstrates the key concept which is the focus of this book: The individual biocompatibility of a material should be fully evaluated before it is placed within a patient.

The ICBM declaration was not entered into lightly. It is the result of the total ICBM Conference which was jointly sponsored by the University of Colorado at Colorado Springs and the Toxic Element Research Foundation during the week of November 5-10, 1988. Dr. Douglas Swartzendruber, an experimental pathologist with Colorado University, and Dr. Hal A. Huggins, General Director of the Toxic Element Research Foundation, were co-chairmen of the Conference.

Twenty-four major speakers representing research efforts from around the world made presentations at the ICBM Conference. Research was presented pertinent to the health risks surrounding the use of restorative materials in medicine and dentistry. Specific topics included toxicology, biocompatibility of materials currently in use, effects by these materials in the brain and nervous system, psychological reactions mediated by materials exposure, immunologic, mutagenic, and teratologic data, as well as risk assessment considerations.

Included among the presenters were the following:

Duane Cutright, DDS, Ph.D., Keynote Speaker
—Former Chief of Oral Pathology for the US Army Institute of Dental Research at the Walter Reed Army Hospital

Louis Chang, Ph.D.
—Director of Interdisciplinary Toxicology and Experimental Pathology, and Professor of Pathology & Toxicology at the University of Arkansas

Klas Nordlind, MD, Ph.D.
—Assistant Professor for the Department of Dermatology at the Karolinska Hospital in Stockholm, Sweden

Magnus Nylander, DDS, Ph.D. Cand.
—Research scientist with the Karolinska Institute in Stockholm, Sweden

Vladmir Bencko, MD, Ph.D., D.Sc.
—Postgraduate School of Medicine in Prague, Czechoslovakia

Max Costa, Ph.D.
—Vice Chairman of the Department of Environmental Medicine at the New York University Medical Center and Professor of Pharmacology at NYU Medical Center

Patrick Exbrayat, DDS, MS, Ph.D. Cand.
—Faculte d'Odontologie de Lyon Department of Dental Materials and Assistant Professor at Lyon University in Lyon, France

Frederick Berglund, MD, Ph.D.
—Research scientist investigating the dangers of materials used in dentistry; Stockholm, Sweden

Mats Hanson, Ph.D.
—Research scientist investigating the dangers of materials used in dentistry; Veberod, Sweden

Horst Poehlmann, MBBS, Ph.D.
—Private medical practice and research in Adelaide, Australia

Joel R. Butler, Ph.D.
—Professor of Psychology at the University of North Texas

Sandra Denton, MD
—Private medical practice in Anchorage, Alaska

Mike Godfrey, MBBS
—Private medical practice and research in Mt. Maunganui, New Zealand

Jean Monro, MD
—Private medical practice and research in London, England

Graeme Ewers, BDSc, Ph.D.
—Adjunct Professor at the University of Western Australia in Perth, Australia

Zane Gard, MD
—Private medical practice in San Diego, California

Paul Slovic, Ph.D.
—President of Decision Research and Former President of the Society for Risk Analysis at the University of Oregon in Eugene, Oregon

Robert Sibelrud, OD, MS, Ph.D. Cand.
—Ph.D. Candidate at Colorado State University and private practice in Fort Collins, CO

Sam Wong, Jr., DDS
—University of Hawaii and private dental practice in Honolulu, Hawaii

Anthony Newbury, MDS, LDS
—Private dental practice in London, England

Douglas Swartzendruber, Ph.D.
—Associate Professor for the Department of Biology at Colorado University at Colorado Springs

Hal A. Huggins, DDS, MS Cand.
—MS Candidate at the University of Colorado at Colorado Springs and General Director of the Toxic Element Research Foundation

Video presentations in absentia and presentation with permission by delegation at the Conference:

Leonard T. Kurlund, MD, Ph.D.
—Department of Health Sciences Research Section of Clinical Epidemiology for the Mayo Clinic in Rochester, MN

Olympio Pinto, DDS, MS
—Private dental practice and research in Rio de Janeiro

Banquet Speaker

In addition Colonel James Irwin, Apollo 15 Astronaut and moon walker was the featured Banquet speaker.

COMPATIBILITY

One of the enlightening events of my studies at UCCS was the discovery that the immune system has a little section reserved for dental materials. That is the area known as toxic events. Toxins usually (although not always) induce a defense reaction from the immune system.

Heavy metal reactions (those to mercury, nickel, beryllium, copper, and even gold) are not immune reactions to the metals themselves. Metallic ions are too small to elicit a response. They react by combining with a resident protein known as "self", or a normal part of your body, and form a protein-metal compound known as a hapten. The immune system identifies this hapten as "non-self", and sets into motion an action to destroy the "non-self". The non-self is really you with a Halloween mask on, but the immune system has a poor sense of humor and kills the cell anyway. This is known as an auto-immune response. Your immune system is killing off your own cells.

Auto-immune diseases are usually of diffuse or unknown origin and do not readily respond to normal medical remedies. Examples are arthritis, multiple sclerosis, systemic lupus erythematosus, and even diabetes. Some of the symptoms may be controlled by drugs, but nothing really makes the disease go away. Nothing, that is, except the occasional removal of the cause. Removal of dental fillings has frequently created a positive response toward reducing the damage from these diseases.

So what is safe? In 1985 I assumed many non-mercury containing materials were safe. At the University we began to test various dental materials. In my office we continued these principles and currently test over 400 dental materials for immune reactivity. It is not surprising that the components of dental silver-mercury amalgam are immune reactive. The percentages surprised me a bit. Today sophisticated highly controlled immune testing gives us the story of how many materials *you* might react to and which ones might be relatively safe. Look at these figures from a study of over 700 patients.

Amalgam Component	Percent of 700 people reactive
Mercury	90.30%
Copper	87.50%
Tin	56.25%
Silver	45.23%
Zinc	83.06%

Amazing? Shocking? Surprising? Safe at any speed? With this amount of immune reactivity potential, and in these days of AIDS fear, is it ethical to place amalgam in people? With mercury's published potential for birth defects, is it moral to punish dentists who refuse to place amalgam in pregnant females? Or non-pregnant? Do males count?

What about the non-amalgam fillings — the composites? Are they safe? Many react in over 50% of those 700 people, and one of the most popular "plastic" fillings shows immune reactivity in over 90% of the population.

What are we doing about it? We test every mercury toxic patient before amalgam removal to assure patients and ourselves that we are using "state of the art" methods of determining biocompatibility to combat the effects of "state of the art" high copper amalgams.

What else? We helped sponsor and underwrite the International Conference on Biocompatibility of Materials (ICBM). It was attended by researchers, physicians and dentists from 13 nations. For a small donation (your choice) to ICBM, at our address, you too can have a 10 page write-up of abstracts of the 22 speakers from 9 countries who high-lighted the program. Proceedings of the Conference are also available from Life Sciences Press in Tacoma (206-272-0530). The conference was held at the Broadmoor Hotel where our international guests were shown what western hospitality can be. Success of the conference will be measured by how many days it takes to eliminate toxic substances from the practice of dentistry. Until then, we continue to test patients (you too, if you like) to find the least offensive materials for your immune system.

UPDATE ON THE PATCH TEST

When I first started working with the mercury patch test I had an idea that mercury was bad, and that there was a percentage of the population greater than zero that reacted to it. I suspected 20% might, but knew I could easily be off 10% either way. Well, I was right. I was off. After doing several hundred patch tests, I found close to 90% of the population had *systemic* reactions. That meant changes in blood pressure, pulse, temperature, while only 30 some percent showed "redness" at the site. Redness was the classical determinant of reactions. After a few courses toward my Masters at the University of Colorado I found out why the differences in reaction.

Skin patch tests determine reactivity from the allergy section of the immune system. That's called an IgE reaction. The reactions mercury was eliciting were the "heavy" reactions relating to autoimmune diseases like multiple sclerosis, lupus erythematosus, and epilepsy. These are from a different part of the immune system by the names of IgM, IgA, and IgG. What this says is that mercury creates much more serious problems than a skin rash.

As we began to see patients with more severe diseases we found one thing to be quite predictable. If the patient had a serious problem, I could turn it on full bore by placing a mercury patch on their arm. We also found people abusing the test. One doctor placed a patch at 4:30 Friday afternoon and left town. By his return Monday morning the patient had been hospitalized, the highway patrol had found me in Colorado, and corrective measures had been initiated. (Remove the patch.)

Many such events taught me that a great number of people are reactive to low doses of mercury exposure. It also taught me that if evidence indicated the patient or I thought a patient might be reactive, the patch testing created a 90% chance of sending them through a torture chamber. We had our patients wait in the office for at least one hour after a patch was placed. After seeing such immediate reactions time after time, I became convinced that many more people were sensitive than I ever guessed, and that patch testing was an unnecessary event any more.

Looking back I would conclude the patch test events finally convinced me of the magnitude of the problem. It was then that I began to concentrate more on helping afflicted patients than in proving that mercury was a poison.

I have not used a patch test in 3 years. I probably never will again. My education in that area is complete.

UPDATE ON CHELATION

There have been a lot of changes in attitude toward Chelation Therapy during the past 4 years. Mostly mine. I was burned on chelation therapy a decade ago by trying to help people recover from what I felt were overdoses of therapy. Today's chelation therapist is much more scientifically oriented and some physicians, like Sandra Denton, M.D., have designed chelation programs specifically for dental patients. Dr. Denton has directed chelation activities that I have observed and I have found them to greatly benefit patients, especially during the amalgam removal procedures.

As in the days of old, I don't feel that gallons of chelation are necessary for dental patients, but a few treatments given during the actual removal procedures, or within a few hours afterward, have demonstrated immediate beneficial effects for those patients.

BUBBLE-OPERATORY

In 1973 I quit placing amalgam fillings. Patient protection? Sure that was a big concern, but I didn't want the daily personal exposure either. My mercury toxic mind and I then continued cutting out old silver mercury amalgams for eleven more years not once thinking that I was taking a shower bath in mercury mist several hours every day.

Read the research by Duane Cutright, DDS. Ph.D. in this book. His article on increases in mercury levels in the brain, heart, liver, and kidney after 10 minute exposures to cutting amalgam started me thinking about a safe dental operatory. After a 6 year gestation period, we gave birth to the first prototype of a dental operatory safe for the patient, doctor and assistant.

Since fillings generate electrical current and all electricity has some effect on the body, we decided to attempt to build an electrically neutral room. We started with a Faraday Cage. This is a fine wire mesh encasing the walls and ceilings that is attached to gorunding rods reaching several meters into the soil. I learned a lot about Faraday Cages *after* this was built, but, after all, it is a prototype, isn't it? Prototype? That's a place to learn before they write the rules. You are limited by your imagination and creativity, but not by what people say can't work. Next we added an electronic mercury particle and vapor removing device and two high powered air filters with a combination of filtrates I researched and designed. The corners and floor to ceiling angles were rounded for better control of air flow, hence the name "Bubble Op" was coined to describe the bubble shaped operatory. Dialysis tubing replaced normal plastic tubing, a cannister assembly for water delivery, and non-out-gassing materials were used for floor, cabinets, and walls.

Paints were tested with a mercury vapor detector to make sure we did not have an unknown source of mercury. Air mercury vapor tests and paticulate counts showed that we had good control over the air. Mercury vapor during active procedures dropped from 880 micrograms per cubic meter of air without the system functioning to 0.000 when it was fully functional.

Would I change anything? You bet. As well as this unit functions, I have already thought of further refinements. I am convinced that dentistry can be accomplished without exposing the patient or personnel to unnecessary toxic chemicals. The future is wide open.

WHAT IS MERCURY TOXICITY?

Am I mercury toxic? Can you test my mercury level? Just what is mercury toxicity anyway? These are common and confusing questions. Mercury attacks many systems in the body. If it attacked just one, like the polio virus or measles virus do, it would be quite easy to identify. The diagnosis of mercury toxicity is based on both the number of changes and the degree of these changes. White blood cells usually increase as a response to the introduction of amalgam. If these cells go up from 5000 count to 7000 count, this is not especially noteable. If the count goes from 5000 to 50,000, then we are talking about leukemia. That is quite noteable. The white cell count bears much more weight in diagnosis at 50,000 than 7,000. Many measurable areas can be affected by mercury. Excerpting from our 1989 edition of the Applications Textbook, here are some examples of the mental gymnastics involved in generating a diagnosis:

Consider:

> White cells above 7500 or below 4500
> Hematocrit above 50% or below 40%
> Lymphocytes above 2800 or below 1800
> Serum total protein above 7.5 g% or below 6.4 g%
> Serum triglycerides above 150 mg.%
> BUN above 18 or below 12 mg%
> Hair Nickel above 1.5 ppm
> Hair Mercury above 1.5 ppm or below 0.4 ppm
> Hair Aluminum above 15 ppm
> Hair Manganese below 0.3 ppm
> Immune reactions to Aluminum, Nickel, Mercury, Copper, and Gold
> Oxyhemoglobin below 55% saturation
> Carboxyhemoglobin above 2.5% saturation
> Presence of root canal treated teeth
> Grouping of symptoms
> Presence of both amalgam and gold
> Magnitude and polarity of electrical current
> T-subset and DNA analysis

This is just a partial list of potentially affected areas. Add to this, the intensity and direction of each reaction and it is obvious that diagnosis of mercury toxicity becomes a Professional Judgement Call. Since each of these reactions potentially affects several others, it becomes increasingly more important to rely upon professional judgement than a single test result.

CHAPTER 1

Amalgam and Its Potential For Destruction

"I've got a pain in my chest."
"Calm down. It's just that you're uptight."
"It makes me breathe faster."
"That's just because you are frightened being in the dental office."
"I've never been frightened before."
"Maybe it's a reaction to the nitrous oxide, but you just had a few whiffs."
"I know. I didn't like the feeling it gave me."
"Many uptight patients feel that way about it."

What's the use. He just doesn't understand. I'll just be still. .

She sat back in the dental chair, resolved to make it through what was really a minor session for three "pit" fillings. It didn't take long. But something was wrong.

That night she began to breathe faster. She was actually hyperventillating. She had heard if it, and was now experiencing it. "It" just came on. There was no reason. She couldn't control it. She had thought that people who experienced it were weak, kooks, had a screw loose somewhere. Then the anxiety hit and hit hard! Why? There was nothing to be afraid of. Panic . . . Blur . . . the emergency room. This was to be the first of dozens of emergency room visits yet to come.

She had a problem — get a check-up: "You're O.K."

The heart is beating funny — go to a cardiologist: "You're O.K."

The pain in the belly is getting worse — go to an internist: "You're O.K., but let's put you in the hospital and run some tests."

Eight days later came the pronouncement. The final diagnosis came after x-rays, probing fingers and an increasing feeling of "fading away." And what was the reason for all these problems?

"NERVES"

She was back home now, and the chest pains were getting severe. She was sure she was going to die. More trips to the emergency room. More hospital tests. More specialists. Then, when all else fails, the psychiatrist, the psychologist, the ministry and finally, the institution.

"No! I won't put my daughter into an asylum. She's not crazy!"

Six months of "pilgrimage" from doctor to doctor (more than 50 in all) lead to what could have been the final verdict: "Lock her up." A frustrated mother, daughter and family. Religion had become their only tangible reality.

You don't just lock up a winner! Her mother told me she had been the most popular girl in her class. A cheerleader. She had been a good student. She had been a happy, charismatic kid exuding love and friendship, an outstanding child!

Yes, my mother loves me too, I thought to myself, as I looked at the pimple-faced, quivering pile of protoplasm trying to claw her heart out of her chest. I certainly didn't see what "mother" described. I couldn't help but feel compassion for this 17-year-old girl who had "been the rounds."

What chance did I have? I had never seen anything like this in dental school! Nor in my 17 years of practice. Compassion melted into another emotion — anger. Is this another case of mercury toxicity? Is this another human being destroyed by one of nature's most insidious poisons? I had no way of knowing, but no time to worry.

We drew blood. The analysis didn't say anything to me. It would today, but in 1979 it looked "normal".

I felt the hair stand up on my arms, then my neck, then my legs. Tears came to my eyes. That was not unusual anymore. I probably went ten years without crying until I got into mercury toxicity diagnosis. Now it was common. My personnel laughed now because they knew I was going to launch into a plan of action that would disrupt the schedule. They didn't mind because they enjoyed the successes. We all hated the failures, but neither happened unless we tried.

Tears used to bother me. Now they don't. They are part compassion, part appreciation for being given the chance to participate in this field and part anger. Anger toward a few men who are just defending their own reputations, and the reputation of an organization. Men who fear for their jobs, fear for their credibility. Fear moves them to deny the existence of people like this girl and all the others that we see on a daily basis.

2

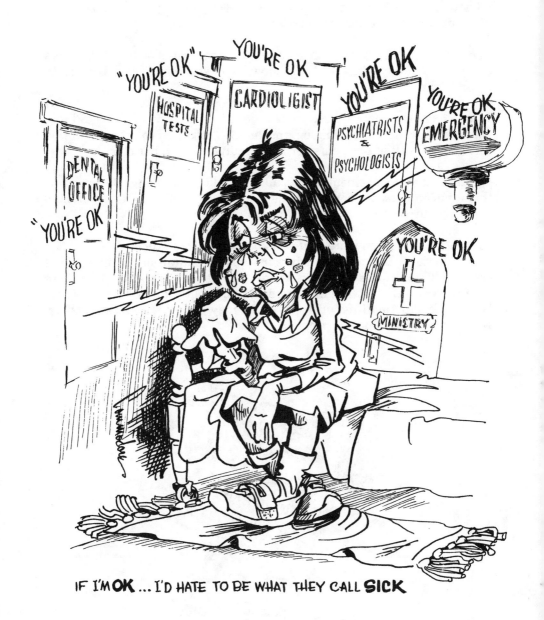

IF I'M **OK** ... I'D HATE TO BE WHAT THEY CALL **SICK**

"O.K. I'll do it."

All it took was 30 minutes to remove six tiny fillings. I didn't know the intricacies of patient protection that we teach now. I just whipped those little amalgams out and put plastic in.

The next three days she went through the open gates of Hell both ways many times a day. With today's knowledge, she would not have had to endure that.

In two days the severe chest pains stopped. In four days she could join her friends for the first time in months. She returned to school, did two semester's work in one semester and graduated with her class.

Graduation announcements don't all mean the same thing. So close was this division between commencement and termination. Six tiny fillings made the difference.

Dramatic? Yes. Even more so if you knew the *whole* story. Unusual? No. Unfortunately. Mercury silently slips out of dental silver fillings and creates all kinds of havoc daily. *All* kinds of havoc? Yes and that's where the problem comes in. Each of us reacts differently to mercury toxicity. We get sent to ten different doctors who may not even know each other. It's a complex diagnostic problem.

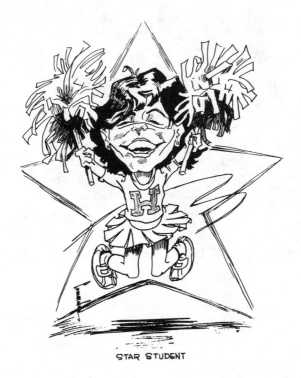

STAR STUDENT

4

"How often does she have seizures like this?"

"Every 15 minutes."

"How long have they been going on?"

"Since October . . . two months. But we could see it coming on in August."

"What happened in August?"

"She had two tiny fillings placed. That's why we're here. She's had $8000 worth of testing at the finest hospital in Denver under one of the best neurologists."

"What do they suggest?"

"That she be put in an institution and both her mother and I undergo psychotherapy."

"How did you find out about me?"

"A lady I met in a health food store told me about her daughter who was having chest pains. They wanted to put her in an institution too. Do you remember her?"

Do I remember . . .

Is this another case of mercury toxicity? The goose bumps, the tears, the anger, the excitement. What if it works?

This child couldn't stand by herself. Couldn't walk. She could just barely think. She had been a straight A student and now this eleven-year-old girl would take an average of 90 seconds to answer the simplest addition problems.

"I want you for my Christmas present," I said as I disrupted the schedule again. Not only mine, but that of my wife as well. With the serious problems I need her to assist me. I can think to her. I don't always have time to find the words that bring the right instrument into my hand at the right instant.

We had 15 minutes between seizures to give anesthetic on both sides, place the rubber dam, get the amalgam out and place new mercury-free fillings. We did it in 14 minutes. Then it hit. She had a violent seizure right in the dental chair. This chair had metal parts. Sharon put her hands on the child's forehead to hold her head in the headrest. Her father

5

sat on her right leg and I sat on the left. Another assistant draped herself across the waist. All of us were thrown up and down like we were on a bucking bronc. We were a combined weight of over 650 pounds and yet we were tossed into the air like rag dolls.

I wonder what the American Dental Association would think about this one, I remember thinking.

It was December 19th. I wanted her well as my Christmas present. Christmas held a special meaning for me. I had told many dental groups who heard my lectures on mercury toxicity, "Send me a Christmas card. I'm going to have mercury eliminated from dentistry by Christmas." That was Christmas of '82. I didn't get any Christmas cards.

On December 25th she woke up. The numbness in her body was gone. Her brain was clear. She got out of bed and walked *downstairs* by herself!

There were no more seizures. The next spring we videotaped her running the 100 yard dash in 14.8 seconds.

I later had a chance to hear a reaction to her improvement from the American Dental Association (ADA). Their official comment to a Florida newspaper was, "We are not impressed." Later they were reported to say that we faked the videotape.

These two stories are true ones, but they could still be used as scripts for horror movies. We're often asked why no one else sees these horror stories. Well, they do. They are seen by other dentists and by other professionals as well. Clinical ecologists see them all the time but are only just beginning to understand the implications of mercury toxicity.

We were instructed recently by a very astute Ph.D. (a professor of statistics) that we must be extremely cautious in our association of "causes and effects". We were told that unless we have *valid* statistical studies we can't make our basic assumption: if we take out amalgams and the patient's symptoms go away, then the problem was caused by the fillings.

Statisticians disagree. We were chastised for forty-five minutes because it would be impossible for us as clinicians to set up a valid study. Even statisticians have a difficult time agreeing upon whether a given study is valid or not. The implication here, of course, is that we don't have degrees in statistics, so we can't possibly be correct when we notice that the hundreds of patients treated by amalgam removal get well.

There seems to be a double standard here. Though *we* are told not to make unsubstantiated comments, it's fine for the ADA to do so. The

ADA has made the statement many times that there is no more of a health problem among dental personnel than there is in the general public. We found an article in the June 1976 *Journal of the American Dental Association* (JADA for short), Vol. 92. The ADA quotes this portion frequently: " . . . no substantial evidence indicates that mercury intoxication is a significant problem among U.S. dental personnel." Insurance companies who have corresponded with us seem to disagree with them. By the way, the next sentence is conspicuously missing from the ADA quotations: "However, to date, there have been no large-scale studies on which to rest such a conclusion."

We are often asked why the majority of dentistry does not embrace our philosophy of treatment and "approve" our work. We have tried over and over again to make excuses for our parent organization, but we are unable to do so any longer. Other concerned dentists have appealed to the ADA through a conservative approach, discussing literature references and giving good recommendations which would allow those who control the ADA to save face.

One good example of this approach was seen as the National Institute of Dental Research/American Dental Association co-sponsored Workshop in July, 1984. The workshop was ostensibly held for the purpose of discussing the effects of various materials used in dentistry upon the health of patients. Research was to be initiated if any of these materials (nickel, mercury, beryllium and others) were suggested to create toxic reactions.

The ADA has turned deaf ears to all of us, patients included. The politicians who control the ADA and who never see dental patients (some aren't even dentists!) have covered up the problem long enough. We are no longer able to make excuses for their obviously inaccurate and misleading statements.

Their conclusions and recommendations at the Workshop on Biocompatibility of Dental Materials were written *prior* to our presentation at that workshop. Though asked to present *only* clinical observations (not statistical or scientific documentation) we were severely criticized for failure to present documentation. It was as if the hundreds of hours spent in preparation for that presentation were wasted.

It is with anger and frustration at being unable to get the ADA to even *recognize* the problem that we are turning to you, the American Public. We have already been criticized for this move. But we are doing it because we fear that too many of you will become ill waiting for the dental and medical "establishments" to do their research. *Recommendations* have been made by the ADA, but this means nothing has been initiated

7

yet. We feel it is your right to know what can happen if mercury amalgam is placed in your mouth or in your family's mouths.

It is our desire that this book be able to arm you, the lay public, with the knowledge you need to protect your health. We will try not to get too technical in the main body of the book. We will discuss first the history behind our work. Then we will describe the problem in full as we see it. Finally, we will discuss our treatment plan.

It is also our desire that our words be read and digested by the dental profession, a group of dedicated, caring individuals who will be needed desperately by those of you with mercury toxicity problems. For our fellow professionals and interested lay persons we have included in the end matter of the book a number of appendices. Here you will find numerous case histories of mercury toxicity, excerpts from pertinent articles in the dental and medical literature with our comments; the entire text of an article co-authored with Dr. O.F. Pinto, the true mentor of awareness of mercury toxicity; and the text of our presentation to the National Institute of Dental Research (NIDR)/American Dental Association Workshop on Biocompatibility of Dental Materials, July 11-13, 1984.

We expect you to have a good understanding of the depth of the problem after reading this book. And we expect to be able to give hope to those of you who have been told for so long that your problems are "all in your head."

Are our two initial stories isolated cases? Not by any means. We see patients with chronic fatigue, multiple sclerosis, depression leading to irritability leading to suicidal thoughts. We see allergies, chest pains, arthritis and scores more. We've been accused of "selling snake oil" by saying that these are all related and that we have an answer which helps.

But the answer is there. Mercury toxicity can do all this — all this and more to the susceptible patient. We estimate that more than 20 percent of the population is affected by mercury toxicity sufficiently to hinder their lives. Our estimate is based upon the number of patients we see as well as the number of patients who are seen across the country by other dentists and physicians.

As you read this book, you'll feel the anger that we feel on a daily basis when we see patients suffer. They shouldn't have to suffer. We hope to make you angry, too. The efforts you make in getting your dentist to understand the problem will help to eliminate this poison so that no one has to suffer because of it again.

8

CHAPTER II

The Fight Against Amalgam — Amalgam Wars, I II And III

Mercury is poisonous. Any high school kid knows that! So how is it that our nation's dentists (educated for eight rigorous years beyond high school) can daily, in good conscience, fill their patients' teeth with an amalgam containing approximately 50 percent mercury? It is a question of misinformation combined with misplaced trust.

Dentists have been taught that mercury stays within a filling and does not come out. When a dentist looks to the professional literature for information about mercury he is apt to find statements like this one by the editor of the *Journal of the American Dental Association (JADA)*: "In answer to the question 'Are amalgam fillings hazardous to the patient?' " this comment was made. "The answer is an unqualified NO. Study after study shows the patient undergoes no risk . . . the dentist, yes, but the hazard can be reduced to practically zero." (March 1971) No one is likely to challenge a statement based on "study after study".

Dental journals condense many months of research into a few pages. The dentist can gain years of experience from his technical trade journals. These are refereed journals. This means that experts in the specific subspecialty fields have reviewed and scrutinized the article for truth and honesty. The dentists rely on this integrity and tend to believe without challenge, because dentistry is a highly ethical profession.

Yet, looking back at that *JADA* quotation now, after eleven years of investigation into mercury toxicity, I note that these "studies" were not referenced. In the hundreds of articles we have accumulated on mercury in the body (see appendix B for excerpts from a few), we have not been able to find even one that would support the claim that mercury is harmless to the patient. Nonetheless, the statement has gone unchallenged.

The same issue of the *Journal* contained an article that made a similar claim: "The amount of mercury vapor emitted from an amalgam is undetectable." Again, I now note, no substantiation, just a statement. Information like this tends to lead a dentist into thinking that he is work-

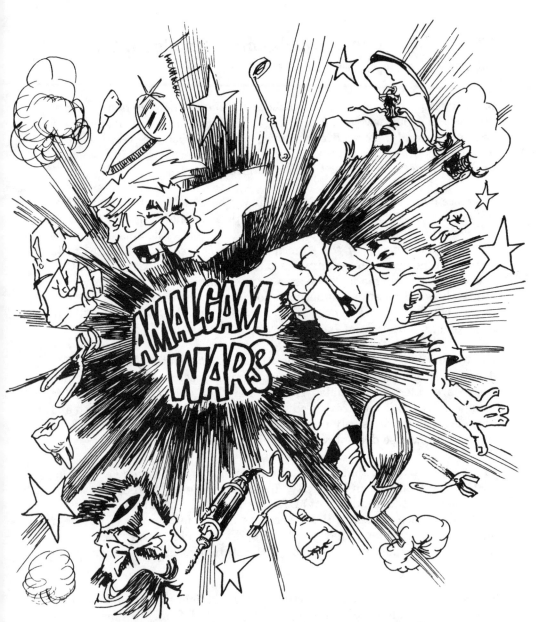

(W)HOLE "**TOOTH**"... NOTHING BUT THE "**TOOTH**"

ing with a material that is unquestionably safe for his patients. It may be dangerous in some forms, yet is certainly safe in the mouth.

To minimize his own risk and the danger to his personnel, the dentist consults articles that recommend a NO TOUCH technique. He is cautioned to avoid touching amalgam with his fingers. Keep scrap amalgam stored in glass containers under glycerine. Keep a lid on it. Get rid of it. Do not store it for long periods of time. Don't have carpeting in the operatory because it harbors mercury vapor. In other words — get rid of scrap amalgam because it is dangerous.

What is scrap amalgam? It's what is left over after the dentist gets through filling your cavity with amalgam. If mercury is so safe in your mouth and so dangerous in the office, then Dr. Jerry Timm was right when he published in the April 26, 1982 issue of the ADA Newsletter the statement that the dental association is telling us that the only safe place to store amalgam is in the mouth.

Amalgam, amalgam, amalgam. If you are like most Americans, you don't really know what amalgam is. Very few lay people (who have amalgams) know that their amalgam or "silver fillings" are mixtures of silver, copper, tin and zinc as a group mixed with an equal amount of mercury. Their silver fillings are actually 50 percent mercury. Fifty percent mercury when placed, that is.

If mercury stays tightly bound in the amalgam compound as dentists are taught, then a five- or ten-year-old filling would still contain 50 percent mercury. They don't. Actual tests show that they contain 25 to 35 percent mercury by that time. Some 20-year-old fillings have less than 5 percent mercury.

Fillings should become less of a problem the older they get, then, shouldn't they? "No," say the allergy doctors. "The more often you are exposed to a substance, the more apt you are to become allergic to it." In addition to this factor, mercury is a cumulative poison.

Is mercury toxicity a new topic? Hardly. It has been debated in dental circles since the 1930's. According to McGehee (1956) and co-authors, amalgam was first introduced in England in 1819 by Bell and later used by Traveau in Paris in 1826.

In the early 1820's, amalgam was introduced into America as a cheaper substitute for the only filling material used at that time — gold. Dentists became quarrelsome about its use right away. Mechanically, the first amalgams were inferior to today's amalgams and tended to expand as they reacted with saliva. Some teeth actually split as the amalgam expanded. You can imagine the pain these people experienced as their fillings slowly split their teeth apart. Dentists who placed gold immediately censured their colleagues for such practices. They also pointed out the poisonous aspects of mercury.

"Amalgam placers" said the "gold placers" were only interested in money and were in essence denying dental services to lower income patients. On the battle waged until it became Amalgam War I. Articles began to appear in the dental research literature. The Amalgam War became an academic conflict. The emotional pitch of the nineteenth-century conflict is evident in some of the titles of the academic onslaughts:

"Death Caused by Swallowing Large Amalgam Filling"
"Diseased Eyes and Amalgam Fillings"
"Mercurial Necrosis Resulting from Amalgam Fillings"
"A Shameful Case of Malpractice (Amalgam Filling)"
"Irritation of the Larynx Caused by an Amalgam Filling"
"Poisoning from Corrosive Sublimate Generated in the Mouth from Amalgam Plugs in the Teeth"
"A Consideration of the Objections Offered by Physicians to Amalgam Fillings"
"Mercurial Poisoning and Amalgam Fillings"
"Case of Deafness Probably Caused by Amalgam Fillings"
"Injurious Effects of Amalgam"
"Salivation Produced by Mixing Amalgams in the Hand"
"The Itinerant Amalgam Peddlers"
"Amalgam and Kindred Poisons"
"In View of the Recent Investigations, Has Amalgam Been a Blessing or Curse to Humanity?"
"Oral Electricity and the New Departure (Amalgam)"
"Amalgam Filling Causing Acid Taste"
"The Amalgam Fraud"
"Death From an Amalgam Plug"
"Acute Mania Attributed to an Amalgam Filling"
"The Amalgam Question Again — Its Moral Aspect"
"The Poisonous Effects of Amalgam Fillings"

The dental community became polarized into two camps: those who abhorred amalgam and those who advertised it heavily. Irreconcilable differences undermined the foundation of the National Association of Dental Surgeons, and soon dentistry was without an organization.

A few years later a new organization came into existence. The American Dental Association. It endorsed amalgam and grew to become the ADA of today. It still endorses amalgam, but the old Amalgam War is rekindling.

Meanwhile, an intermediate European skirmish began in the 1920s and was led by one of Germany's most outstanding chemists, Dr. Alfred Stock. He published over 30 articles condemning the use of amalgam. His research methods were surprisingly accurate; they rival the most sophisticated techniques of the 80s. He was gaining headway in drawing attention to diseases that were stimulated by mercury leaching out of fillings. After he became suspicious that mercury was the source of his own myriad of medical problems, he had his amalgams removed. When his medical problems improved as a result of amalgam removal, he then "treated" many friends by encouraging them to have their amalgams removed also. Finally the dental community of Europe gave credence to his findings and he gained academic as well as public support.

Stock became somewhat discouraged and lost the drive in his research when his laboratory and most of his records were destroyed by a bombing raid in World War II. World War II ended Amalgam War II, and Dr. Stock died in near obscurity.

The war lay dormant.

Very little was heard about amalgam for three decades. I was certainly unaware of mercury hazards in the late 50s and early 60s during my dental training. As students, we mixed eight parts mercury with five parts powdered metal, placed the soupy mixture in a *squeeze cloth* and twisted the cloth to "express" out the excess mercury. The excess mercury would fall onto a metal tray and roll into a reservoir of mercury sitting open in the clinic. As we squeezed out the excess mercury, some of the liquid mercury would hit the metal tray and splash onto the floor. Thousands of tiny droplets would scatter across the clinic floor to find new homes in cracks, equipment and shoes. According to figures published later, only 20 percent of the mercury dispensed left the clinic in patient's mouths.

Mexico City brought about my initiation to the problem. I had spoken before the International Academy of Gnathology on how balancing body chemistry (my primary subject of interest at that time) could increase bone density and reduce gum disease. I pointed out several abnormalities of blood chemistry that would not respond to treatment, and casually mentioned that I did not know why.

That void of knowledge was soon filled as Dr. Olympio Pinto of Rio de Janeiro came up to me after my presentation. "Those nonresponsive areas are easy to explain," he began. "They are due to sulfhydryl blockage by mercury leaching out of amalgam fillings." I wasn't too sure what sulfhydryl blockage was, but I was secure in my belief that amalgam was a stable compound. In fact, not just a compound, an *alloy*. It sounded so much more prestigious to place an alloy than an amalgam that I had always used the term alloy.

"Why, mercury doesn't come out of amalgam," I began and then muttered something about alpha phase, gamma phase and other terms I mimicked from my dental school professors. I could see that I wasn't having much impact on this man from Brazil. How was I to know that I was talking to one of the world's authorities on mercury toxicity?

The next two hours were intense. Olympio's parents were both dentists. His father had attended a conference in the 1920's in which a speaker had condemned mercury. The elder Pinto remembered this a while later when he was asked to treat the gums of a child dying of leukemia. Her biggest complaint was that her gums hurt. The elder Pinto removed her amalgams quietly, and the terminally ill child responded within a few days. *Spontaneous remission* announced the medical profession. Pinto responded by telling the physician he had removed the amalgams. There is a pecking order today in the health professions. There was then too. He was academically whiplashed and made to feel inferior and foolish. Standard procedure. Pinto quietly replaced an amalgam, then told the doctor to watch for a recurrence of the leukemia the next day. Recurrence happened. He removed it, of course, and the child recovered again.

I was in shock. "It's got to be a coincidence," was my first scientific reaction.

"Then there was the case of Hodgkin's Disease," continued Olympio.

"Hodgkins?" I retorted. "Wait a minute. You're talking about heavies. Medical diseases! Real diseases! Not allergic reactions."

Olympio quietly proceeded with diseases and dates. "This type of leukemia was not noted until 1832, a short time after amalgam was introduced in the area where the disease was discovered. The first amalgam to be placed in a Negro was in 1904. Sickle cell anemia was first noted in 1906."

"But pathologists weren't very smart then," I challenged. Later I found that some of the most brilliant pathologists the world has ever known were alive then. I also found that sickle cells are not difficult to identify.

By the end of the two hours I had made a solemn personal vow. I would never mention these findings to a dental group. I kept that vow with an agonized, haunting feeling that some day the secret would slip out. It did. Three weeks later while I was lecturing to an especially cordial group in the South, I let it slip.

"Would you fellows like to hear something really way out?" I heard myself say. As I spoke, one member of the audience paled. He had had Hodgkin's Disease and had been terminal. His amalgams were removed

14

during a dental study club educational project and his diagnosed Hodgkins had gone into *spontaneous remission.* That was about 12 years prior.

I felt a cold chill spread from my neck outward to my arms, legs, feet and hands. My eyes became cloudy. I had just experienced the birth of Amalgam War III.

The years from 1973 through 1979 were frustrating years. Success would peek through the muddled chemistries about once every three to six months. Then it would disappear with no hope of ever reappearing. No predictability. Far more failure than success met my attempts to be another Pinto. I continued to mention the problem as I lectured on body chemistry. Everyone thought it was interesting, but in private would let me in on certain "secrets": If mercury were really a problem, the ADA would have found it out a hundred years ago.

The FDA would certainly not allow such a substance to be used. They protect our health.

Congress would legislate sanctions against mercury if it were a problem.

The AMA monitors anything related to health. They would surely spot any problems that might have arisen.

O.K., O.K.! We are protected. But how do you explain the one case in ten or fifteen of mine that *has* responded? Spontaneous remission!

I wanted to quit. I prefer success to failure and certainly the scales were biased. I lost more than I won. My colleagues were kind, but not supportive. They kept giving advice. "You're going to get your license lifted." "You're practicing medicine without a license." "You're wrong."

The successes were uplifting, but the failures made me feel that I was wrong. The time spent, the financial drain, the emotional drain and the friendships that dissolved were easy to put on the scales. I was teaching how to balance chemistry, while I was living a totally unbalanced life. I've been asked many times, "Why did you continue?" I have an honest answer. I don't know.

The question arose, was I practicing medicine? My thought was that if I were practicing medicine, then the inverse would apply. Medical doctors would be doing what I was doing for these patients. That certainly didn't match. The medical profession was not even suggesting a connection between mercury and these diseases. They relied upon the ADA's stance that mercury in dental fillings is safe.

I took this problem to a board certified forensic pathologist. This brand of medical doctor is the supreme court justice of medicine. I could drop this in *his* lap. Dr. David Bowerman was presented with the problem of the decade. If mercury is causing all these medical diseases, then *you* get in there and clean it up.

"If dentistry has created a problem, it is the responsibility of dentistry to investigate and resolve the problem," quoth the pathologist. Somehow I felt the meaning of the word **Nevermore**.

I was alone again.

Then came 1979. That was the year they began to fit. No wonder I hadn't seen the big picture. I had had only a fraction of the pieces to the mercury puzzle. I met a giant. Jess Clifford. He taught me about cell morphology. Under Hoffman contrast microscopy, red and white blood cells began to take on personalities and meaning.

Then I found by accident that some fillings have negative electrical current. Electrical current had been known since 1880, but what did *negative* current mean? (I'll get to that later.) This discovery was probably the single most important factor in the quantum leap that our success ratio took from 1979 through 1984.

A host of other factors were seen in patients suffering with mercury toxicity. Electrocardiogram changes appeared. Then I could detect mercury vapor by placing an industrial meter into people's mouths. Changes occurred in the retina of the eye. They could even be photographed. Dormant chemistry changes could be stimulated by getting rid of the amalgam. New relationships emerged in the chemistries. If "X" goes up, "Y" goes down. And at long last the original sentence by Olympio was explained. Sulfhydryl groups appeared. Dr. Al Belian first told me about sulfhydryl groups in hemoglobin. A whole new battle plan emerged with the help of Dr. Belian, Dr. Bowerman and one of Olympio's video tapes of live blood cells in action. After all the parts were assembled, we had unlocked the primary problem that plagued the majority of my patients — chronic fatigue.

Exciting years! New diseases responded to amalgam removal. Success was up to 50, 60 and 70 percent. Elation over patient improvements was evident in my whole staff. Phone calls were approaching 20 to 30 a day. The mail was heavier. Interest was expanding. Work days were becoming longer. Financial productivity was dropping due to requests from the public and professionals that I attempted to satisfy. Accounting figures began to show red ink. Then came the supreme blow.

I had lectured at most of the major national dental meetings including the national ADA program. I had spent 60 to 100 days a year lecturing to dental groups in the U.S., Canada, Mexico and Europe. My ego was fed by comments like, "That's the first time I sat through an all day lecture without falling asleep." "You really give us things we can go home and use." "I've never felt so good since I adopted your program." I was convinced that teaching was my best suit. By this time my wife Sharon had joined me on the lecture tours. We complemented each other. I taught theory and philosophy and got their attention. She could make them understand the procedures and teach them how to start putting our information into their practice. Together we made a good teaching team. We enjoyed lecturing and were well received. Then it happened. Organized dentistry sent out the edict, "If you have Huggins on your program, no continuing education credit will be given to the doctors in attendance." We were dead in the water.

Our lecture schedule dropped to zero. I had cut back my dental practice to one day a month. We were devoting 26 to 28 days a month to answering letters and calls and to seeing one or two mercury toxic patients per day. The books were redder. I had to accept living expenses from my father and from Sharon's premarital funds. Then a kind researcher, Wilmer Eames, from Denver published an article implying that I was gouging the public by placing gold where it wasn't necessary. His assumption and public statement was that we were reaping enormous profits. Shades of Amalgam War I.

Well, at least I haven't lost any weight and even though my car is aging, it can still break the speed limit. But I have something that no salary can match. I feel an inner glow of satisfaction when I think of our successful cases.

During this 1979 through 1984 period there was another fire smoldering within me. A smoldering fire of discontent that was bred from observations of "terminal" diseases that were spontaneously remissing. They were remissing consistently on the fourth or fifth day of treatment. Remarkable that spontaneity was so predictable.

Sarcasm became my major weapon. The academic world wanted double blind studies. No one seemed to care about recovered patients. Those patients were only anecdotes and therefore of little or no value. I didn't have a Ph.D. so therefore I was of little or no value. I felt that they suffered from *paralysis through analysis*. They wanted us to replace amalgam in the recovered patients and duplicate the disease again. I mentioned this to some of the patients. Funny they all had the same instructions for me to give the scientific community. They could go to a warm place.

Smoldering became glowing, became burning discontent and turned to an internal inferno at the active lack of interest in ever investigating the issue. Sharon and I vowed that we would make exposure of mercury's potential for destruction the prime objective of our lives.

If I folded financially, Sharon would accept it. My father didn't comment. He knew that we were committed. He checks on me daily to see how the war is going. Somehow I missed Korea and Vietnam, but I earned my stripes in the Amalgam War III.

After eleven years of ignoring the issue, Dr. Joyce Reese of the National Institute of Dental Research (NIDR) called me. They were co-sponsoring a workshop on metal toxicity with the ADA to determine whether mercury is a topic worthy of investigation.

My thinking had to be direct and organized at the NIDR workshop. I was asked to present patient observations — no double blind studies were expected. Dr. Reese, program chairman for the workshop, was very kind in assuring me that it is the job of NIDR to determine research maneuvers — not mine. She indicated that clinical observations were of value. That was an attitude I had never seen from the academic world.

I wanted to talk about multiple sclerosis, show videotapes of the epileptic before and after treatment, show videotaped interviews. Then I remembered the three researchers who had just visited my office.

"Do you want to see the videotapes?" I had offered.

"No," was the cool response, "We are only interested in research."

These people were also to be at the NIDR/ADA workshop. I was about to be suckered into my favorite topic, "Look what can be done for people!" It would be best that my clinical observations be limited to chemistries. That's probably what Dr. Reese meant. If I spoke about patients, the term anecdote would surface again, and the Amalgam War would grow cold for another generation.

Bottom line is the popular buzz word of today, and it applies to many more things than accounting. What is my bottom line? *Mercury is a problem.* What would I have to do to plant that idea? We have given three-day seminars on the subject of mercury alone. Here we would have only 45 minutes. I had better be organized (not my major suit). Then a thought came to mind which became the outline for the presentation.

In order for mercury to be a problem, it would have to
1. come out of the filling
2. form a compound that is toxic
3. form sufficient quantity of this compound to produce disease and
4. demonstrate remission of the symptoms upon amalgam removal.

Having stated the problem, I would have to explain how to diagnose and treat the mercury-toxic patient. But first I had to break down the inertia of the ages that assumed that mercury was "tightly bound in an intermetallic compound."

So Sharon and I worked hard at getting ready for the workshop. I labored over what turned out to be a sixty-page manuscript (with references) and she spent long, grueling hours getting it all typed and corrected. At the same time we were trying to manage our day-to-day business and practice affairs, and continue to see patients. We spent hours going over the speech, determining the exact amount of time I could spend on each topic. (Sharon held up cards to keep me on time at the presentation.)

We labored over every word, trying to say everything in a manner so as to be forceful and effective without "treading on toes". We tried to put everything together in such a way as to facilitate the right decisions without anyone having to admit former mistakes.

At last we were ready. Somewhat apprehensively we left for Chicago — bolstered by encouraging words from colleagues and friends but knowing what the outcome could be.

We sat through the first day's presentations rather ignored by the majority of those in attendance. Few wanted to admit they knew us; fewer wanted to be seen talking to us.

We listened to the questions asked of the other clinicians by the audience. All seemed to be professional — certainly nothing for us to be concerned about. The clinicians for that day seemed to be presenting good information but with weak conclusions. But after all, this was the academic world, and their jobs would depend upon their not "rocking the boat."

My time to speak came, and nervously I approached the podium. My opening comments were light (supposed to be humorous) but no one laughed. No one even cracked a smile. I could tell that "hostile audience" was an understatement.

I concluded my presentation. The questions began. The first hangman didn't really want to ask a question. He wanted to disprove a statement I had made. The second wanted only to dress me down in public and vent his anger against me. He never got around to asking a question either.

The third accused me of interfering with his doctor/patient relationship with a patient I had never seen, never spoken with and never corresponded with. Again, no question! The fourth demanded that I describe all of my "entrepreneurial interests" and financial affairs. From there they got worse. Knowing that my position would be precarious (the only one advocating abolition of amalgam), the petite Dr. Reese had jokingly promised to be my "body guard" throughout the proceedings. Where was she when the stones were being thrown? Sitting with the ADA.

It would have been worth all the insults and criticisms had the recommendation of the workshop been to discontinue the use of amalgam until further studies could prove its safety. But the spokesmen did no such thing. Their recommendations boiled down to meaning that no action was being taken because no documentation had been presented to show problems. These conclusions were seen in typed form three hours *before* I presented our material. Their statements are presented along with the text of our paper in appendix D.

The next day, one of the doctors in the audience (he was not a clinician and prefers to remain unnamed) stood up and gave the following speech for the workshop record:

> "Advocates of dental mercury amalgam fillings claim that the safety of those fillings has been scientifically proven and documented numerous times and that it has been continuously reaffirmed over the 150 years of its use.

> "Let me relate my experiences in this regard. Upon being informed by Dr. Hal Huggins in September of 1981 that mercury was not locked into the filling alloy and that the release of mercury could constitute a potential health hazard to the patient, I decided to investigate the matter for myself.

> "I first turned to the oral pathology and dental materials textbooks. *Skinner's Science of Dental Materials* by R.W. Phillips stated that dental amalgam should not be placed in contact with gold restorations in the oral cavity. In *A Textbook of Oral Pathology* by Schafer, Hines and Levy I found this statement: 'A toxic reaction from absorption of mercury in dental amalgam has been reported on a number of occasions.'

"Shocked by these findings, I next turned to pathology, physiology, pharmacology, chemistry and other textbooks and was further alarmed after learning the effects of mercury and its compounds on the human body.

"I wrote the American Dental Association and requested the actual *Primary* research establishing the safety of mercury amalgams in patients. The ADA sent one secondary research article [this means that it only quotes the primary article which is based on actual research] and a form letter stating the ADA position. On it were listed eight references: one was the secondary article they sent, one was a U.S. Government statistical report on dentists, two were primary research papers indicating that mercury is released from amalgams and four were primary research papers based on urine mercury measurements. [The ADA now acknowledges that urine mercury measurements do NOT correlate to the toxic effects of mercury.]

"I then called the ADA and specifically requested the primary research establishing the safety of mercury amalgams in patients. I was told that none was available and was referred to the National Institute of Dental Research (NIDR) of the NIH.

"The same request was presented to the NIDR — same result — none available. The NIDR said that the responsibility for establishing the safety of dental mercury amalgam belonged to the Dental Materials Division of the National Bureau of Standards.

"The same request was then presented to that organization. I was told that there was plenty of research available investigating potential risk to dentists from the use of mercury, but there was none available relating to patient risk because in 1957 Frykholm proved that dental mercury did not present a risk to patients. [Frykholm utilized experimental techniques and equipment, including urine mercury measurements now known to be inadequate.]

"I then turned to the research literature myself. I have now accumulated, read and documented over 600 references on mercury and dental amalgam. I am absolutely convinced that the use of mercury amalgam in dentistry does constitute a potential health risk to patients."

One member of the audience thanked us for "stepping into the lion's den". This was after the workshop was over and when no one else was around. It sounded nice, but somehow it didn't soothe the ache of knowing that still nothing would be done. How many more lives will have to be ruined before they listen?

We returned to Colorado, temporarily down emotionally but still determined. After much soul-searching, Sharon and I agreed to use this book to say everything that needs to be said to you — the public — regardless of the outcome.

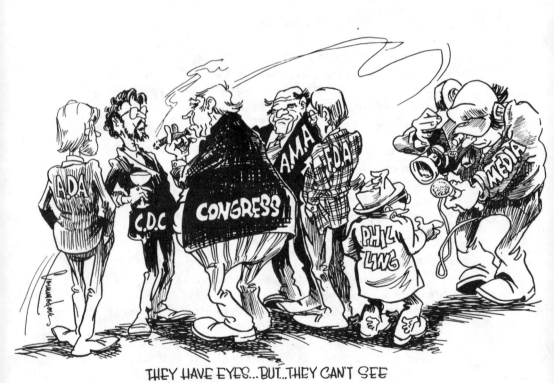

THEY HAVE EYES...BUT...THEY CAN'T SEE

CHAPTER III

Dynamics Of Mercury

Mercury DOES Come Out of Fillings!

Before we can discuss how to solve the mercury problem, we must establish that there *is* a problem. This we will accomplish by meeting these challenges that you will remember from the last chapter:

1. Does mercury come out of the filling?
2. Does it form a compound that is toxic?
3. Does it form enough of this compound to produce illness? and
4. Can a reduction of illness upon amalgam removal be demonstrated?

Let's consider the first question. Amalgam is a mixture of mercury (Hg), silver (Ag), copper (Cu), tin (Sn) and zinc (Zn). Mercury is the biggest portion (around 50 percent) and zinc the least (around 1 percent). Each manufacturer has a different formula, so the other metals vary in composition. Copper can vary from 3 to 30 percent and silver from 15 to 30 percent, while tin is usually around 10 percent.

Chemical reactions normally take place between two types of chemicals. Those with positive charges react with those having negative charges. A common example of this is when positively charged hydrogen (H+) reacts with negatively charged oxygen (O=) to produce H_2O or water. All the components of dental amalgam are positively charged. The question is, do they actually "react" together or do they just form a mixture that hardens?

Actually many chemical reactions occur. More than a dozen compounds exist in amalgam. Copper joins with oxygen, mercury, chlorine and sulfur (from foods); silver joins with tin, mercury, chlorine, copper and combinations of all other metals present. Actual chemical formulas are listed in the manuscript (appendix D).

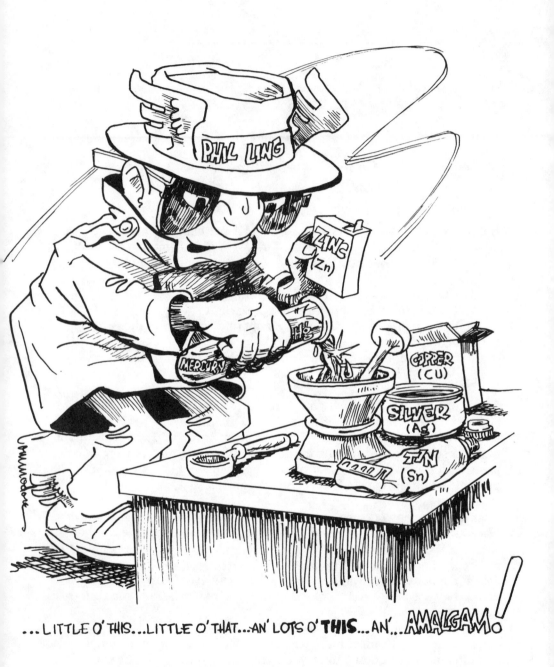

...LITTLE O' THIS...LITTLE O' THAT...AN' LOTS O' **THIS**...AN'...AMALGAM!

It is difficult to design an experiment that would produce all these potential chemical reactions in a laboratory, because the mouth contains a complex chemical environment that has yet to be duplicated in a test tube. Temperature changes; cigarette smoking; chewing gum; chewing ice; drinking hot coffee; eating salty, acidic or bland foods; ingesting sugars, and chewing tobacco as well as having bacteria and other fillings in the mouth produce a constantly changing environment. Such mechanical and chemical stressors can be duplicated for no more than a few minutes at a time.

Electrical current produced in the mouth is probably the single most damaging stressor, yet very little is known about it. J.J.R. Patrick was the first to describe electrical current in the mouth back in 1880. He called it oral galvanism.

In 1979, nearly 100 years later, we bought an electrical current measuring device — an ammeter similar to those used in drug stores to check batteries — and started touching fillings. My goodness! There *was* electrical current! As we touched fillings we suspected that electricity moved in several directions in the mouth. Touching two fillings on the right side, then two on the left side and then one on each side didn't result in readings one would predict mathematically. Current had to be going through the head.

From courses in physics, we knew that if several steel ball bearings touched each other, electrical current could travel in one end and out the other end — no matter how many ball bearings there were. As long as they touched.

When we touched a filling it discharged (like a flash camera in principle) and the meter gave us a reading. If we touched it again a few seconds later, the charge was much less. Touching it again was practically not measurable. Given 10 to 20 minutes the charge would build up again.

Combining our discharge observations with the steel ball bearing information, it would stand to reason that if four teeth had four fillings touching each other, a discharge of the first one would discharge all of them. Sounded great. The only thing is, it didn't work that way. Each filling discharged independently. That meant that the charge had to be traveling down the tooth and into the body, not from filling to filling.

Let a gold crown be placed beside an amalgam filling, though, and all kinds of electrical fury was unleashed. Through a European research effort (Wranglen, 1983) we learned that an electrical path exists between the filling itself and the natural fluids in the tooth *under* the filling. We were reminded of that famous traffic nightmare in Rome where about six streets converge into a circular intersection with no traffic lights.

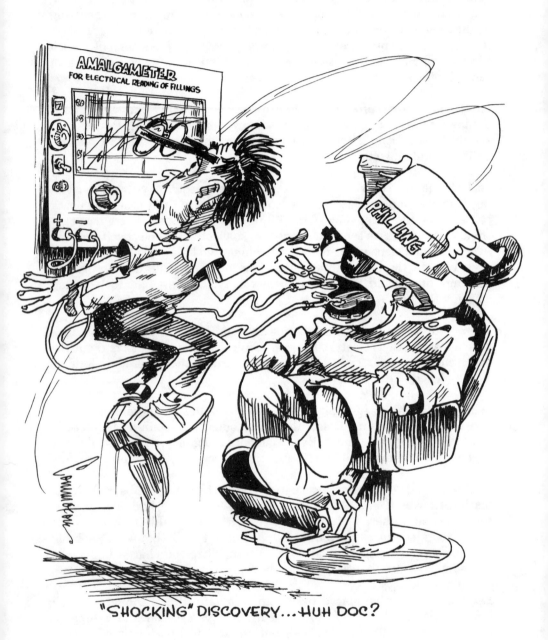

"SHOCKING" DISCOVERY...HUH DOC?

We began to look for more detail about electrical pathways generated in connection with fillings.

We learned that there are two types of electrical activity on the surface of a filling. One is like a standard battery. Two different metals in an electrolyte (solution that can conduct electricity) will produce a current (flow of electrons). This is called a *bimetallic cell.* (The term "cell" refers to a minute area that produces electrical activity.) The other cell which exists on a filling has an anything but obvious name — *differential aeration cell.* Sounds like something you might use in the kitchen after cutting onions! This refers to electrical activity that exists between two areas of saliva containing different amounts of oxygen. An area of saliva which is low in oxygen (closest to the filling) can react with oxygen-rich surface saliva exposed to your breath.

There is a common denominator among electrical cells. They all have both positive and negative parts. The negative is called the anode, or sacrifice anode. (Now, you don't get something for nothing. So when you get electrical current, a chemical compound has to be lost. Hence the term "sacrifice" anode.) Something is "given off" there. Actually in an amalgam, just about any metal can be "given off". But our concern is that the largest volume "sacrificed" at the anode is mercury. Sacrificed so that *you* can absorb it.

Chemically it looks like mercury is able to come out of a filling. But isn't there an easy way to just measure it? Yes, it so happens that there is.

One day a psychologist was in our office interviewing patients after their amalgams were removed. His statement at that time was that *people process thought differently when they no longer have mercury in their mouths.* At one point in time during the interviews he laughed, and we noticed that he had a mouth full of amalgams. We had just borrowed a Bacharach Mercury Detector from the Department of Public Health to test our office. Could there be enough vapor coming off all those fillings to be detected by an industrial meter? Hummmmm . . . Probably not, but then one never knows unless he tries!

We asked him to open his mouth, placed the tube over a filling and all watched in stupefied silence as the needle went to 10, then 20, then 30 and then 50 mcg/M³ — *past OSHA's maximum to 60-70-80 and finally to 90 mcg/M³. At a level of 50 mcg/M³, OSHA fines offices $10,000 and closes their doors. Here was a university professor minding his own business, yet contaminating his own body with toxic mercury every time he inhaled or ate. Shouldn't OSHA fine him, too?*

We knew mercury came out of fillings, but had no idea it came out *that* fast. We had read Dr. Wilmer Eames in the ADA Journal proclaiming that amalgam elicits high vapor levels for only a few seconds. We had read other ADA articles saying "mercury vapor over amalgam is undectable". Undetectable? How? By not looking!

We began to test routinely for mercury vapor above fillings and found everything from zero readings to more than double OSHA's maximum limit. One patient, after chewing gum for two minutes, exhibited a level of 300 mcg/M^3 over his fillings.[1]

Other researchers are finding these levels now. Independently, Dr. Gay (1979) and Dr. Svare (1981) registered high breath concentrations of mercury, especially after their subjects had been chewing gum.

Measuring vapor was a simple enough test, but what about analyzing old fillings? Is that hard to do? Not if you have the proper equipment. Jaro Pleva of Sweden (1983) analyzed a five-year-old filling and found it contained 27 percent mercury. Compare this with the average 50 percent mercury in new fillings and you can see that nearly half the mercury had leached out in five years.

We did tests on some amalgams of known age and found two that had 36 percent mercury. One was seven years old, the other eleven years old. It was interesting to note that the seven-year-old amalgam had nearly double the electrical current found in the one which was eleven years old. This suggests that mercury loss is probably a function of the intensity of the electrical current in the filling.

As if this isn't bad enough, there is a new hazard on the scene. High copper amalgam. Several decades ago, copper amalgam was outlawed due to its toxicity. Even as recently as five years ago, its cytotoxic properties (ability to cause death to the body's cells) were being discussed in the *Journal of Dental Research* (see appendix B). After testing several different types of amalgam, researchers found that, "Copper amalgam yielded the most intense cytotoxicity of them all." The conclusion of the study reads this way: "Furthermore, necessity for long-term biocompatibility tests was also stressed, since the restorative materials are kept in the mouth for quite a long period once inserted."

Now the copper amalgam is back. Not only is it back, but it is the fastest selling amalgam on the market today!

What's bad about it as far as we are concerned is that when a patient reacts to a high copper amalgam, his chances of recovery are much lower than if the older amalgam of the early 70s had been used. This is especially true in cases of neurological damage.

We had observed this, but it wasn't until 1983 that we got a hint as to why this was happening. An article appeared in the *Scandanavian Journal of Dental Research* showing the difference between conventional amalgam and the new "high copper" (30 percent copper) amalgams. The authors showed that the high copper amalgams were so much more chemically reactive that they gave off mercury *50 times faster* than conventional (3-6 percent copper) amalgams. Maybe that's why they are so damaging. In our opinion high copper amalgam certainly should be banned immediately if our protective agencies have any concern about mercury toxicity from fillings.

You don't have to let a dentist place high copper amalgam in your mouth. You don't have to let him put *any* mercury in your molars.

You particularly don't need mercury if you have any tendency toward gum disease. A Georgetown University study published in 1978 described a patient with advanced gum disease. As amalgams were removed by quadrant (a fourth of the mouth at a time), the gum disease healed in that quadrant while continuing in quadrants where amalgam remained. After the final amalgam was removed, her whole mouth was healed of gum disease and had remained healthy for two years after amalgam removal.

There's not much room for doubt that mercury does come out of fillings. It is easy to prove and easy to duplicate these tests.

Corrosion DOES Produce a Toxic Compound

What happens to mercury when it does come out of a filling? The next challenge concerns its toxicity.

Does corrosion really have to produce a toxic compound? Plain mercury when uncombined with anything is poisonous. Isn't that bad enough? Well, it probably is but it just so happens that mercury is highly reactive chemically. It likes to combine with biological tissue. In the mouth, mercury has the ability to combine with a carbon-hydrogen compound called a methyl group. When mercury combines with methyl groups it is called *methyl mercury.*

Talk about toxic! Methyl mercury is 100 times more toxic than plain, elemental mercury. Methyl mercury is especially toxic to the brain and nerve tissue which may explain amalgam's relationship to multiple sclerosis, epilepsy and emotional disturbances.

Jaro Pleva wrote in 1983, "A few months after the final dental treatment I was surprised by strong, unexplainable symptoms. I woke up in the nights with intense anxiety and irregular heartbeat and each time, for a few minutes, I thought that these were the last minutes of my life. At the same time, other acute symptoms increased very much. A state of indescribable tiredness, stress and anxiety was constantly present. To perform simple tasks, to join discussions, to think, talk and to be social required considerable effort."

As if that weren't bad enough, methyl mercury can cause birth defects by altering the body's chromosomes. A drug called Colchicine is the standard of comparison for chemicals that produce birth defects and chromosomal damage. It is the strongest drug known for producing genetic problems. Methyl mercury is *1000 times more toxic genetically than Colchicine.*

Now how do you feel about running out to get your teeth filled with mercury when you find that you are pregnant? Well, there's the placental barrier. That should protect the little tyke. Studies have shown that the red blood cells (good mercury carriers) of the unborn infant contain 30 percent *more* mercury than its mother's.

Let's get a little more detailed here. *Saying* that methyl mercury is formed is one thing, but *substantiating* it is another. Here is an in-office explanation of the parts of the puzzle that are documented in the literature plus a part that we have discovered in our work, as yet unpublished.

A man named Heintze did research at the University of Lund in Sweden to show that the process of methylation (combining a methyl group to a metal) can take place in the mouth. His 1983 research showed that there is a bacterium in the mouth that has a highly developed ability to methylate mercury. This bug is called *Streptococcus mutans.* It is the bug that is associated with dental decay according to current thought. *Strep mutans* is in everyone's mouths; you don't just catch it.

What a situation! A bacterium that can produce deadly methyl mercury lives on the filling that gives off mercury. Here's where our discovery may play a role. We have noted that people who have the more severe neurological diseases like MS, epilepsy, depression and suicidal thoughts tend to have fillings with negative electrical current. Going back to Heintze's research, the bacterium he used as a "control" in determining how powerful *Strep mutans* is works best in an environment with a very low oxygen level. If it is possible that low oxygen levels (called low oxygen tension) in saliva can improve *Strep mutans*' ability to methylate, then could it be that negative electrical current on a filling might produce low oxygen tension in the saliva covering it? If it does, then there could be more methyl mercury and thus more of the diseases we observe in conjunction with negative fillings. This certainly is worthy of a bit of further research.

In answer to the challenge then, it is fairly obvious that mercury *does* form a toxic compound when it is given off the fillings during the corrosion process. If one of the world's most dreaded toxic compounds can be formed in the mouth and inhaled or absorbed into the body, is dentistry justified in submitting trusting patients to it on a routine basis just because it is easy to handle and is cheap? Is it necessary that the filling material be able to outlive the patient?

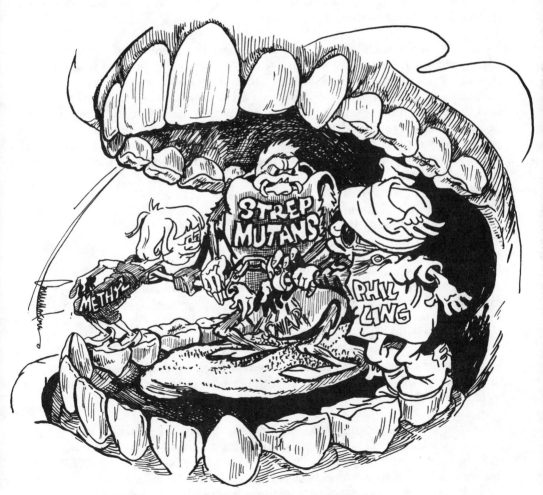

WATCH YOUR MOUTH

There IS Sufficient Toxic Material To Cause Disease

The next challenge involves quantity. Can enough mercury escape from amalgam to produce a toxic level? Based on an article by Thomas Eyl, M.D., (1970) levels should not exceed 100 parts per billion. That would correspond to a daily dose not to exceed 100 mcg.

Other researchers find problems at even lower levels. Sharma and Obersteiner (1981) found that a few micrograms severely disturb cellular function. They also found that mercury inhibits growth of nerve fibers at much lower concentrations. "A few" sounds to us like 1 to 10 micrograms (mcg) at most. Again, this would tend to suggest that women during pregnancy should not have amalgam in their mouths at all — much less have a fresh batch placed.

Neither of us want to be pregnant, but we are both jealous of the pregnant female. In the field of health, we think *everyone* should be treated like a pregnant female. Coffee is fine — unless you are a pregnant female. Take this drug twice daily — unless you are a pregnant female. Mercury is O.K. to be around — unless you are a pregnant female. Why can't we all be treated like a pregnant female? We all want our cells to function properly. We want our nerve fibers to grow and conduct impulses properly. How come they get all the TLC, while we non-pregos get the axe?

Back to how much is safe. Dr. Alfred Stock of Germany (1939) and Dr. Trachktenberg of Russia (1969) identified toxicity at very low levels. Stock found problems if the air contains 2 mcg/M^3 and Trachktenberg found problems at 1 mcg/M^3.

Whether we use 1, 2, 5 or 10 micrograms as safe limits really doesn't seem to matter. Radics, a European researcher found that the average mouthful of amalgam can produce 150 micrograms of mercury in 24 hours. This is an average, of course, and can be reduced by chewing ice or increased by drinking hot coffee or chewing gum.

How much mercury does it take? Is there enough coming out of a filling to create a problem? Come walk in our shoes for a day or two and there would be no doubt in your mind.

From the practical standpoint, we have seen reversal of really severe disease by removal of one to three small fillings. One 16-year-old boy was so fatigued he could only go to school on a part time basis. One small filling (called a pit filling) stood between him and full teenage activity. He could keep up with his peers within three weeks of amalgam removal.

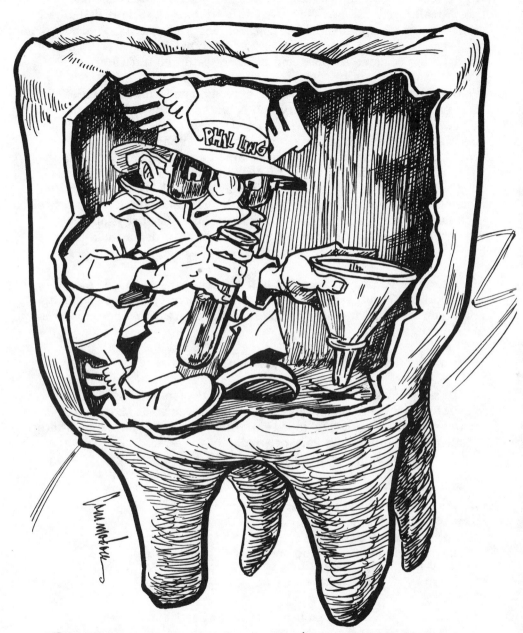

FUNNELING MERCURIAL ILLS INTO THE SYSTEM

An 11-year-old girl was having seizures every 15 minutes. She had only three small "pit" fillings. Neurologists were baffled. She had the best diagnostic work-ups available. But no one thought of "harmless" amalgam fillings as a potential cause. Within five days of amalgam removal, her seizures stopped and have not returned in two years.

We were recently sent a copy of a list of recommendations to dentists for their protection against mercury and scrap amalgam. It was published by the Council on Dental Materials and Devices of the American Dental Association. It warns of the severe hazards of the vapor coming from scrap amalgam. Remember that scrap amalgam is the part of the filling left over when you have a filling placed but not all of the amalgam is used. The scrap is put into a can or a box and "saved" to be returned for reclamation. The proper handling of this dangerous material which emits such harmful vapors is considered such a problem that it is also recommended that dental students be taught these hazards as well. There is one article to this effect in appendix B.

Since scrap amalgam is the other half of the amalgam that is placed in your tooth, it sounds reasonable that these recommendations should apply to you as well. After all, you have the identical "hazardous" material in your mouth.

Here are the Council's recommendations:

1. Store mercury in unbreakable, tightly sealed containers.
2. Perform all operations involving mercury over areas that have impervious and suitably lipped surfaces so as to confine and facilitate recovery of spilled mercury or amalgam.
3. Clean up any spilled mercury immediately. Droplets may be picked up with narrow bore tubing connected (via a wash-bottle trap) to the low-volume aspirator of the dental unit.
4. Use tightly closed capsules during amalgamation. (This means while it is being mixed.)
5. Use a *no-touch* technique for handling the amalgam.
6. Salvage all amalgam scrap and store it under water.
7. Work in well-ventilated spaces.
8. Avoid carpeting dental operatories as decontamination is not possible.
9. Eliminate the use of mercury-containing solutions.
10. Avoid heating mercury or amalgam.
11. Use water spray and suction when grinding dental amalgam.
12. Use conventional dental amalgam compacting procedures, manual and mechanical, but do not use ultrasonic amalgam condensors.
13. Perform yearly mercury determinations on all personnel regularly employed in dental offices.

14. Have periodic mercury vapor level determinations made in operatories.
15. Alert all personnel involved in handling of mercury, especially during training or indoctrination periods, of the potential hazard of mercury vapor and the necessity for observing good mercury hygiene practices.

Now let's apply these recommendations to the (scrap) amalgam in your mouth:
1. Use a no touch technique. (Keep your tongue off of it.)
2. Store it in an unbreakable, tightly sealed container. (Put your head in a box.)
3. Store (scrap) amalgam under water. (Keep your tongue off of it with your head in an unbreakable box submerged in water.)
4. Work in well-ventilated spaces. (Keep air circulating in your mouth while keeping your tongue off the [scrap] amalgam with your head in an unbreakable box submerged in water.)
5. Avoid heating amalgam. (Don't drink hot coffee or eat Mexican food while circulating air in your mouth with your tongue off the amalgam and your head in an unbreakable box submerged in water.)

It makes you wonder, doesn't it? Why is the ADA more concerned about scrap amalgam than it is about the amalgam in your mouth?

Is there enough vapor and toxic material given off to cause problems? Yes!

Disease CAN Be Reversed By Sequential Amalgam Removal

Can sequential amalgam removal produce remission of disease symptoms? Yes, it can. And what's more, the procedure can cause improvements in the blood tests, CBC, urinary excretion of mercury, blood pressure and body temperature. With more sophisticated testing we can detect improvements in electrocardiograms, vision and retinal changes and circulation to the brain (as seen in thermography).

West and Todd (1957) state: "The toxicity of mercuric ions is largely due to their combination with the sulfhydryl group (SH) of enzymes with resulting inactivation. Thus it is seen that the physician is constantly confronted with abnormal states which are the result of, or attended by, changes in the chemical reactions within tissues."

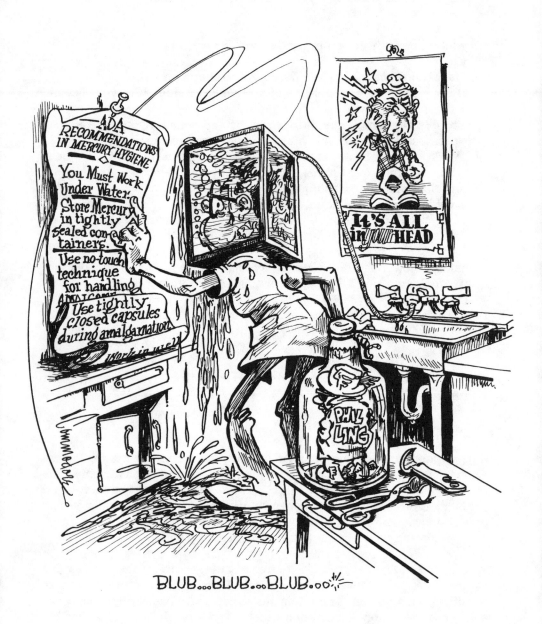

According to the same authors: "Certain heavy metals are classed as enzyme poisons, although they would better be classed as inactivators or inhibitors, since many of the reactions are *reversible!* Mercury, silver and gold are examples."

Do the diseases improve 100 percent of the time? No, they don't. The percentage is much higher now than it used to be. Our success rate now is closer to 80 percent as opposed to the 10 percent we used to see before we understood the importance of electrical current and the need for supplementation during the procedure.

We have seen many diseases respond to one extent or another and have grouped them into six general categories:

>Neurological
>Cardiovascular
>Collagen
>Immunological
>Allergy
>Miscellaneous

Neurological

The diseases in this category are of two types: those which affect motor function and those which are emotional. The largest part of our practice involves MS (multiple sclerosis) patients. The next largest is patients with suicidal tendencies followed closely by those suffering fatigue. Why do we see so many MS patients, while the MS Society denies amalgam as one of the initiating factors? Refer to appendix B for a discussion of the article "Comparative Epidemiology of Multiple Sclerosis and Dental Caries" for further information.

"Wheelchairs are for old people, not me!" This thirty-two year old patient struggled through the resistance of uncooperative muscles held back by multiple sclerosis. She got out of the chair. Within a short time she was back in it again. Through determination and a will to win, she got out again.

That's when we saw her. One thing about MS patients — at least the ones we see — is that they are gutsy. The upsetting thing about this patient was that she had *no* negative fillings. She had about a dozen positive ones, but no negatives. She had been diagnosed as having MS by a neurologist 12 years prior.

When she was getting out of the dental chair she glared at us and pointedly asked, "Do you ski?"

"Yep, thirty years worth," was the reply.

"Next year I'm going to race you on the ski slopes, and I'm going to whip you!"

"You find a ski slope, I'll race you and Sharon will capture it on film."

A little over a year later, the two of us rode the lift and Sharon had to lug the video equipment up the slopes through the trees to get a good shot. (I should have consulted Sharon first before promising to videotape the event!) What did we capture on tape? I was thoroughly whipped!

Three weeks later this excited ex-MS patient called to say that she had just skied the "Plunge" — the most difficult slope in North America. We happened to have an MS patient in the office at that time, so we told him the good news.

"Next year I'm going to ski with both of you."

That started the MS Ski Team. We now have eight struggling MS'ers who could care less about the disease per se. They want on the '85 Team. Bless them.

The same day we got a letter from the MS society. They informed us that a search of the literature proves that amalgam has nothing to do with MS. Bless them.

Depression and suicidal thoughts seem to be a natural part of mercury toxicity. While it is true that depression often follows a prolonged illness, this is not usually the type of depression seen in the mercury toxic patient. The depression has a sudden onset and usually is not caused by anything in particular. Many times it overtakes the patients when everything is going great. And yet, physicians who are unable to find an organic cause and make a diagnosis refer the patient to a psychiatrist for help because "it's all in your head."

The suicidal patient is very special to us. We do all we can to assure these patients that they are not immoral for having such thoughts. This is a unique problem as seen in the mercury toxic patient because the thoughts seem reasonable to them. It is not a matter of right and wrong for them. As one patient described the sensation, "It is a go-with-the-flow feeling." The decision as to whether they should put a knife through their chest is no more important than the one as to whether to tie their shoe.

This presents a real dilemma to those patients with strong religious backgrounds. All religions teach that suicide is a mortal sin. The stronger the religious attitude, the more guilty the patient feels about these uncontrollable thoughts. One such patient's story is detailed in appendix A.

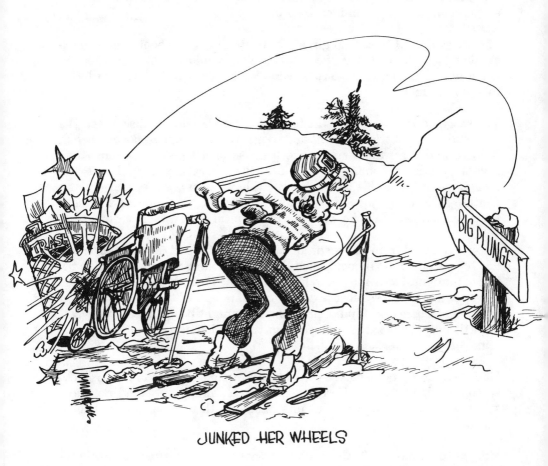

JUNKED HER WHEELS

Cardiovascular

In this category we see such mild conditions as high or low blood pressure and fast pulse rates. We also see more severe conditions like tachycardia (this is where the heart races over 200 beats per minute), angina and severe but unidentified chest pains.

The story of the 17-year-old girl at the beginning of the book is a good example of the unidentified chest pains. They could not be measured by hospital instrumentation so they were "all in her head". Does that begin to sound familiar?

The story of another of our dental patients tells how we discovered the importance of electrical current and sequential amalgam removal. He had been retired from military service because of a heart condition. After several years of coming to us for dental treatment, he broke the amalgams in two of his teeth. As would have been the procedure in any dental office, we removed the broken amalgams and prepared the teeth for crowns. That night he went to the hospital with a tachycardia.

He was released from the hospital seven days later and returned to the office for his crowns. We mentioned that we felt there was a connection between his dental treatment and his trip to the hospital. We removed three more fillings at his request because he wanted all of the amalgam out if they could cause that kind of problem. That night he again had tachycardia. His hospital stay was shorter that time. When the last amalgam was removed, there were no problems.

Had we understood negative current at that time, we would have removed the amalgams in a different sequence. He probably would not have spent time in the hospital. But unfortunately this is the way we had to learn.

How is this man now? Although he is not completely free of heart problems, his physicians no longer recommend the bypass surgery or the pacemaker that he had been advised to have. He follows the dietary principles as explained in Chapter V and has follow-up testing done fairly regularly to make certain that his supplementation is correct.

Collagen

The most common disease in this group is arthritis, while others include Lupus erythematosis and scleroderma. The severity of the arthritis can range from mild swelling and stiffness, to crippling. Diet and supplementation play an especially big role for the arthritic. Citrus juices and many grains, including wheat, must be avoided almost entirely. And caffeine must definitely be out of the diet of the arthritic.

One of our patients demonstrates similarities of diseases and suggests a common denominator. As a professional percussion musician she was devastated to "lose her grip" to arthritis. It was an emotional blow on top of a tentative diagnosis of Lupus erythematosis. The fact that she was now stuttering and having difficulty remembering things compounded her fears of inadequacy in a field where she held a national reputation for excellence.

Here two different diseases in the same category were thought to be her problem.

Negative electrical current was found on some *crowns* in her mouth. They were nickel crowns. Our theory which has been mentioned before is that methyl mercury is more apt to appear in the presence of negative current. Methyl mercury could easily be the common denominator in all her problems. Within two stormy months of ups and downs after amalgam removal, her problems resolved and she is again comfortable in the slot of excellence. Her story is detailed more in appendix A where thorough case histories are discussed.

Immunological

As the name implies, this group of diseases is due to a breakdown in the body's immune system — it's ability to fight disease. Cancers are placed in this category, especially leukemia and Hodgkin's disease. Mononucleosis also belongs in this group.

Leukemia is a cancerous disease in which the bone marrow produces abnormally large numbers of white blood cells. We just recently saw a patient with a white cell count of 235,000 (the medical normal is 5000-10,000). After his amalgams had been out for only 40 hours there was a 60,000 count drop in total white cells. Other highly significant changes in the types of cells being produced to fight the infection in his body occurred during the same two-day period. He had arrived in our office on a Wednesday, certain that he would die of chronic myelogenous leukemia (CML) in three months. He returned to his home four days later, certain that he would live. Was he qualified to make this decision? Yes, he is a physician.

What was his dental condition when he came to us for diagnosis and treatment planning? He had a nickel crown and 21 amalgam fillings.

Twelve of them showed negative current with one as high as -40. Though he was extremely skeptical until the follow-up CBC (complete blood count), *we* knew that we had a good chance of helping him.

We expect to spend a great deal of our energies in the future on leukemia. Concepts like the following description of leukemia by Collins (1959) give us added incentive:

> "Clinical observation of acute leukemia of lymphatic type following immunological procedures started a train of thought which led to the hypothesis that leukemia is an abnormal or pathologically excessive response to an antigen or prolonged antigenic stimulation which may be electively administered or may result from *environmental hazards.*

> "Attempts to transmit leukemia from man to man, even by blood transfusion, have not been successful. This is not surprising if the concept that leukemia is an abnormal response to antigenic stimulation is correct."

Is it possible that the "antigen" is methyl mercury from dental fillings?

Allergy

Though all types of allergies — food and airborne — are seen in the mercury toxic patient, the worst problem we see is the universal reactor. There are an estimated 10,000 such patients in the U.S. today, many without hope of leading a normal life. They are literally allergic to everything in our environment except basics like cotton and wood. Many of them have extremely restricted diets and some can't even be around other people without having severe reactions.

This severity is usually seen in patients who have multiple metals in their mouths — nickel, gold and amalgam. However, we have seen some patients with only amalgam. These patients usually have a long history of small problems which gradually become bigger (often when additional dental work or other exposure to mercury occurs) until they react to everything.

Why would allergies be a part of mercury toxicity? When mercury enters a white blood cell, it causes the cell to produce what is known as aberrant structures. Think of this process as being like a Volkswagon assembly line putting together a Cadillac part along with its parts for a VW bus. When the wrong parts are sent to the Golgi apparatus for assembly within the white blood cell, the "quality control section" recognizes them as aberrant structures. The cell then begins to self-destruct by bringing in water until it bursts.

Inside that cell are hundreds of enzyme packets whose function it is to destroy bacteria and foreign bodies as they are "eaten" by the white cells. This is how the immune system — the white blood cells — protect the body from disease. When the cell ruptures, these enzyme packets are set free in the blood stream to destroy whatever they contact. In simple terms, what we have just described is the allergic reaction.

One such case of severe allergy involves an M.D. Dr. A became allergic to x-ray film and x-ray solution. That wouldn't be such a problem for most of us, but that happened to be his specialty. Soon he was allergic to most foods and chemicals and had a new title — Universal Reactor. He could eat lion, hippopotamus, elephant and snake. Only one food per meal could be tolerated. His weight went from 190 to 120 pounds. His asthma made it impossible to breathe for more than a few minutes without bronchiospasms.

For those of you who are familiar with blood counts, his Eosinophils had hit a record 64 percent recently. They were 46 percent when we saw him. An EOS count of 0 to 2 percent is good, while 10 percent means highly allergic. His wife had to drive him over 2000 miles of back roads at night to get to Colorado Springs. Diesel fumes would send him into bronchiospasms and he couldn't breathe. Airplanes with their jet fuel and cigarette smoke were entirely out of the question.

After the removal of only one-third of the amalgams, his EOS dropped from 46 percent to 2 percent. Four different hospitals were asked to do the count to verify it. They all reported 2 percent. His white cells dropped from 9000 to 5500. On the fourth day we took him out for what we considered the "supreme challenge". Mexican food. In his words, "I tolerated it beautifully."

He gained back 30 pounds, then began to have problems again. A base material called "Dycal" was under many of the fillings. He began to react to that almost as much as to the mercury.

Another trip to the dentist — actually many trips — and now he has all gold fillings. Several other complications set in, but we spoke with him during the writing of this book and he is ready to go back to practice. Will he go back into radiology? No. Preventive medicine and the *real* cause of diseases — mercury toxicity. He has studied much during his convalescence and now has some brand new, exciting ideas to contribute. No more lions, tigers and bears for him now.

Miscellaneous

There are other symptoms and diseases which just don't seem to fit into a specific category. Fatigue falls into this group and is usually seen along with other symptoms. This will be thoroughly addressed in chapter IV so we won't go into detail here.

Another very common problem is that of digestive problems. They can be as mild as indigestion and gas after eating — especially after a protein meal — and as severe as ulcers or Crohn's Disease. They normally involve an inability to properly digest protein. Because protein metabolism is so important to the effectiveness of the immune system and also plays a role in the control of allergies, this particular problem can have far reaching effects.

One of our first considerations in nutritional counseling for the mercury toxic patient involves teaching him or her to eat plenty of protein — preferably animal protein. This also involves the use of digestive enzymes and cutting down on liquids during meals to enhance breakdown of protein in the stomach. This is explained in greater detail in the chapter on nutritional do's and don'ts.

The patient who has problems digesting protein will need more digestive enzymes than other patients during the dental treatment phase. The enzymes taken at mealtime will help digest foods while the ones taken between meals will assist with the globulin stripping as described in Chapter IV.

There are other seemingly unconnected symptoms. If you look at the questionnaire in Chapter IV, you will see the majority of them. But how could so many different problems be caused by mercury and no one have found it out before now? Let Dr. Olympio Pinto describe it to you. Here are some excerpts from his article, "Mercury Poisoning in America" which you'll find printed in its entirety in appendix C.

> "In the fields of the Dental and Medical sciences, due to the progressive deepening and ramification of knowledge, there are no more Dentists or Physicians, but Surgeons, Orthodontists, Prosthodontists, Pathologists, Hematologists, Gastroenterologists, etc., and the men involved in one discipline regard the next discipline as

44

something belonging to his colleague three doors
down the corridor. The so-called General Practitioner is no longer interested in collecting scientific
information, since his field is limited to the surface
of his science. Many times a patient is wrongly referred to a specialist for treatment, and starts an interminable 'pilgrimage', frequently finding the right
man when it is already too late.

"It is interesting to note that the more the patient's
condition aggravates, the closer contact he maintains with the 'specialist' and the more distant he is
from the dentist (either by financial problems or by
the presence of health problems of more urgent
nature). At the time that the patient is referred to
the dentist, most often for complete removal of the
teeth, it is already too late, since the patient's
organism has undergone irreversible pathological
changes".

He also relates for you the relative time of appearance of some of the major diseases as compared to when amalgams were first placed.

"Of course the fact that the most important
diseases have been diagnosed after the appearance
of the amalgam in dentistry is in part due to the fact
that we are becoming better diagnosticians and better diagnostic weapons become more available every
day. However, we should also regard very carefully
any vestige or evidence left whenever we talk in
terms of research, particularly when it is related to
human health.

"According to Goldberg, amalgam was first introduced in the United States in 1825. McGehee
(1956) and co-authors state that the first silver
amalgam is supposed to have been introduced by
Bell of England in 1819 and later used by Traveau in
Paris in 1826.

"In a review of the history of medicine it is recorded
that nephritis (kidney inflammation) was first
recognized in 1827, Hodgkin's disease in 1832,
leukemia in 1845, Addison's disease in 1849, Banti's
disease in 1881, Gaucher's disease in 1882, anorexia
nervosa in 1888, Dercum's disease in 1892, Van

45

Jaksch's anemia in 1890, sickle cell anemia in 1910, chronic monocytic leukemia in 1913, to mention only a few.

"Another curious fact is that the above-mentioned diseases are all of unclear or unknown etiology, presenting at the same time many common symptoms with chronic heavy metal poisoning, as it is the case of a diffuse and irregular osteoporosis of the calvarium (skull) that appear in Hodgkin's disease, sickle cell anemia, leukemia and blood dyscrasias of the childhood."

This may be circumstantial evidence. But we feel that in combination with the reversal of these diseases upon removal of amalgam (seen by many other health professionals as well as in our office), there is more to it than mere circumstance.

Another interesting fact about mercury toxic patients is that their diseases are difficult to diagnose. Most of the serious patients have been to more than 20 different specialists in an effort to get a diagnosis and "cure". They usually are told that "it's all in your head". When this pattern is present and the disease resembles the ones we have described or the symptoms are those as listed in the screening questionnaire (Chapter IV), it is a pretty safe bet that mercury toxicity is involved with the problem.

There is one final factor which we feel must be addressed before we close this chapter. What happens to patients who get well? This sounds like a strange question, but it has great significance.

When chronic or terminal illness strikes a family, emotional and functional adjustments must be made by all the family members. In one case, the wife was stricken with severe fatigue, with allergies, with emotional problems and the husband had to take over her role. He cared for the children as well as her. He washed clothes, cooked the meals, cleaned the house, bought the food — all the things she would have done if she were only well enough. He came to enjoy her total dependence upon him even though it created a hardship for him. The children were a part of this attitude as well.

When the patient began to feel better and began to assume her responsibilities again, the husband became withdrawn and depressed because he no longer felt needed. Professional counseling was necessary to prevent their getting a divorce.

We strongly suggest to our patients that they openly and frankly discuss the possible effects wellness will have upon their family relationship. We hope that if they are warned about the potential problem, they can seek proper help along the road to physical recovery.

Our question remains. Does dentistry have the right to affect the lives of so many people in so many adverse ways? Our answer (to use the words of a former editor of the ADA Journal) is "an unequivocal No"!!!

-----

[1] A government agency called OSHA (Occupational Safety and Hazard Agency) has set limits to mercury exposure that, when exceeded, constitute exposures hazardous to health. At 50 mcg/M^3 (micrograms of mercury per cubic meter of air), OSHA's toxic limit is quite a bit higher than, say, Switzerland's at 10 mcg/M^3. In Russia, Germany and Switzerland mercury toxicity has been found in humans at levels between 10 and 20 mcg/M^3. Some U.S. agencies are now "pushing" for a drop in OSHA's toxicity limit to 25 mcg/M^3.

CHAPTER IV

Diagnostics In Mercury Toxicity

Is it Possible That You Have Mercury Toxicity?

Should everyone run right out and have all his fillings removed? NO!! That's not wise. Not everyone responds with dreaded disease. It isn't necessary to ever have another amalgam placed, but not everyone needs to have their amalgams removed.

Is it *possible* for everyone to have their amalgams removed? We don't think so. We figure that the average dentist can place nine amalgams daily. Out of the 130,000 dentists, let's say 100,000 are in general practice placing amalgams. That's 900,000 amalgams per day being placed. Over a period of years, that adds up to a lot of amalgam out there. When we practiced what is called "wet finger dentistry" (hands-in-the-mouth dentistry), we found that we could average one patient per day doing amalgam removal. One patient per day was average for us. Of course, that included interruptions for telephone calls all day long, so perhaps two patients daily would be a more reasonable rate. That's assuming that no regular patients needed anything done. As much as dentists complain about not having enough to do today, we hardly think they could keep up with replacing 10 percent of your fillings.

Who *does* need amalgam removal? Obviously those of you with problems that have been *shown* to respond to amalgam removal should consider the procedure. Perhaps next on the list should be those with negative fillings, because they are in a profile to develop problems. Last in line would be those people whose other tests (explained later in this chapter) suggest susceptibility to diseases. This basic question of "Who?" stimulated us to develop testing parameters that could separate the sensitive patients from those who are not sensitive. We found one thing right off the bat. There is no one test to distinguish the sensitive from the safe.

There are four ways in which patients may be screened for possible sensitivity to mercury. None of the four can be considered diagnostic in itself. But considered together they can indicate the degree of your sensitivity and help you and your doctor decide whether you should have your amalgams replaced with a non-toxic material.

The four screening measures we currently use are:

1. Symptom questionnaire
2. Electrical reading of the fillings
3. Urine mercury analysis
4. Skin patch testing

There are other screening measures currently being used by other doctors.

The measurement of the amount of mercury vapor coming off a patient's fillings is the foremost of these. While this is interesting and does reconfirm that vapor is given off, it should not be considered as a diagnostic tool. It should not be the sole basis for determining the need to remove amalgam because it does not indicate sensitivity to mercury. It indicates only the patient's exposure to it. It is good as an addition to the other screening procedures.

Symptom Questionnaire

Let's look first at the health or symptom questionnaire. We have included an example of the one we use in our office. We teach other doctors to look for certain indications of sensitivity with this questionnaire. Though there is no specific "rating" system, there are guidelines to use.

Notice that there are different sections to group the similar symptoms under general categories. The mercury toxic (sensitive) patient usually has multiple symptoms in a variety of categories. Seldom do we see the patient who checks only one symptom in each category.

Patients known as universal reactors are those who are allergic to practically everything in our environment. You may have heard of persons who must live in the mountains or away from the city in order to exist. This type of patient will usually check nearly everything on the questionnaire. Are they hypochondriacs? No! They just are so allergic to everything that practically every system in their body is affected. Mercury certainly causes a problem for these patients.

Then there is the patient who checks only one symptom — let's say "frequent headaches" under *Annoying Symptoms*. We always question our patients as to the severity of the symptom. If the headaches come often but are relieved by a couple of aspirin — no big deal. But if the headache is so severe that sight is affected and the patient is rendered nonfunctional — now it does indicate a potential problem with mercury. We had one patient who had been through many neurological work-ups, all sorts of dental and medical treatment including severing several nerves and still had no relief from his headaches. Sleep was possible for only an hour or so at a time. After amalgam removal the headaches were diminished to the extent that sleep was once again possible, and only minor medications were needed for relief.

Look for a moment at all those symptoms listed under *Annoying Symptoms*. They don't seem to be connected do they? Scientific minds look at them and say, "That covers just about every illness known to man" and promptly discount them as not being related to mercury toxicity. However, each one is documented in the literature as being related to mercury toxicity.

How do they relate to each other? They are all symptoms of deficiencies in areas where mercury interferes with enzyme activity. Remember the statement made by Collins about mercury being an inactivator of enzyme systems in the last chapter?

For instance, "ringing in the ears" is related to manganese deficiency. Mercury interferes with manganese metabolism.

"Chronic fatigue" is a result of insufficient oxygen to the cells. Mercury interferes with the ability of hemoglobin to transport oxygen.

"Slow healing" is in part a result of zinc deficiency. Mercury interferes with zinc metabolism.

"Getting up at night to urinate" is a result of insufficient action of the posterior pituitary hormone. Mercury interferes with the production of and the activity of posterior pituitary hormone.

And so on it goes.

Look carefully at the questionnaire to see what symptoms you have. Did you answer "yes" to several of them? Do you feel that you have enough of a problem that it warrants correction?

Have you gone through conventional diagnostic measures to try to correct the problems already and found that they didn't help? Are you like the patient who suffered from severe indigestion including cramping, bloating and gas distension? She went through upper and lower GI x-ray

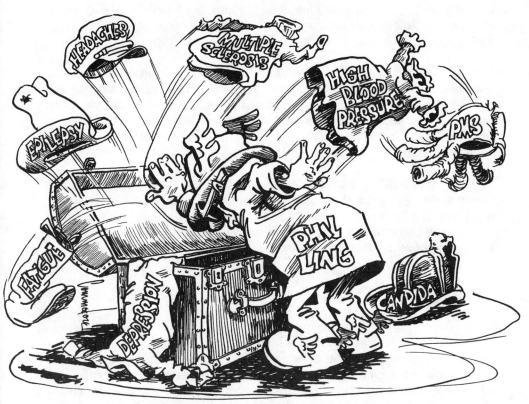

NOT PANDORA'S BOX...BUT THIS TRUNK'LL DO

series (complete with barium enema!) only to find that medically she was "perfectly normal". It was "all in her head" — until her amalgams were removed. The problem cleared up without further treatment and without medication. If this sounds like your story then perhaps you should consider amalgam removal. But remember, the procedure *must* be done in the proper sequence and with proper biochemical coverage to enable your body to excrete the stored mercury. Otherwise, your problems may get no better at all.

Electrical Reading of Fillings

We will only lightly touch upon this subject here because it will be covered in great detail later. But as a screening measure it is excellent.

If you've decided after looking at the symptom questionnaire that you may have a problem, one of the next steps is to have the electrical current on the fillings checked out. This is a very simple procedure. Using an instrument called an Amalgameter, a ground is placed under your tongue and a probe is touched to each tooth which has a filling in it.

If negative electrical current is found, our recommendation is that you should definitely have your fillings replaced. Remember that we see negative current closely associated with neurological problems, both muscular (like MS) and emotional. The more fillings with negative current you have, the greater the probability that your symptoms are caused — at least in part — by mercury toxicity.

If there is no reading with the Amalgameter for a particular filling, the chances are 80 percent that the filling has negative current. Corroded fillings are often hard to get a reading from and must be polished in order to remove the corrosion so that the reading can be taken. Most often, these highly corroded fillings are in this shape because of negative current.

Urine Mercury Analysis

If there's not a dentist near you who has an Amalgameter, another good screening procedure is the measurement of the amount of mercury in your urine. This can be done simply and inexpensively regardless of where you live. So if you aren't fortunate enough to live near a dentist who can guide you toward your decision about your amalgams, you can still find help.

The significance of the urine mercury analysis will be explained thoroughly in the section entitled Urinary Mercury Excretion. At this point we will simply say that the less mercury you have in your urine, the greater your problem with mercury retention toxicity. We are all exposed on a daily basis to pollutants in the air we breathe, the water we drink, and the food we eat. If our bodies are functioning properly, we will eliminate these pollutants. If the cells are not able to get rid of these toxins, expecially mercury, we become toxic. The ADA argues this term "mercury toxic". They prefer to use the term "hypersensitive" to mercury. It sounds so much nicer, doesn't it? But it doesn't really describe the reactions going on in the body.

Toxicity indicates interference with function by a substance which slows biological activity. This is what mercury is doing when it is being stored in the cells. It interferes with mineral and hormone metabolism and enzyme activities. This we call toxicity — not hypersensitivity.

When a low urine mercury is seen, we know that the body is storing the mercury in the cells. Therefore, we must be able to analyze the mercury down to levels as low as 0.1 mcg/L (micrograms of mercury per liter of urine). Most laboratories only measure as low as 20 mcg/L. But in our practice we seldom see levels that high.

If you have answered "yes" to several symptoms and also have a low urine mercury level, again you should consider having your amalgams replaced. Remember that the sequence of replacement and biochemical coverage are extremely important if you wish to get rid of your symptoms.

Skin Patch Test

The last screening measure we will describe is one which is very good and is relatively inexpensive. It was the first method we used and continues to be quite reliable. However, it does have some drawbacks and precautions which should be taken. Here are some things you should know before having this screening procedure — just in case your doctor is not fully aware of them.

Certain patients should *not* have the patch test. Contraindications include:

> Pregnancy
> Seizures — epilepsy
> Severe emotional problems
> Severe multiple sclerosis
> Severe Candidiasis
> Severe heart problems

Mercury passes the placental barrier as mentioned before. Because the absorption of mercury with the patch test is so good, there is a sufficient amount to affect the fetus. For this reason we do not expose our pregnant patients to the patch test as a screening measure. We rely upon the other three methods as indicators of problems. Actually, we only use screening procedures on the pregnant patient if she isn't sure what she wants to do. It is our biased opinion that all mercury should be removed from the mouth of a pregnant patient as soon as possible. It, of course, would be better if it were removed before pregnancy occurs.

As far as all of the rest of the situations are concerned, we'll just say this. We don't put a patch on anyone who has a problem we don't want to see manifested in our office. The purpose of the patch is to determine sensitivity and also to determine which symptoms, if any, are caused by mercury. If a patient's seizures are a result of mercury toxicity, then placement of the patch will bring on a seizure. The same is true for all the other symptoms and disease conditions.

The concentration of the mercury solution used in the patch test was selected because it gives indication of the degree of sensitivity to mercury. Not everyone reacts within the first 24 hours, though everyone will react sooner or later. Those who react within the first hour are the most sensitive and should be considered for amalgam removal before those who react later during the 24-hour period of the test. They are the ones most likely to develop severe health problems.

What constitutes a reaction to the patch? A localized skin reaction is seen in only about 35 percent of all patients tested and is *not* what we look for. We look for systemic reactions. In other words, we are looking for physiological changes, not local reactions. Physiological changes are those in blood pressure, pulse rate and temperature. They can also be an exacerbation or exaggeration of specific symptoms like headaches, fatigue and so forth.

These reactions can occur at any time during which the patch is placed. They can also reoccur if you are exposed to mercury again a short time later after the patch is removed. Please refer to Chapter VI for a list of other ways in which you can be exposed. Be sure to avoid these things for a couple of days after the patch test. Otherwise you could be like the following patient who had a severe reaction to the patch in the first hour.

The patch was removed and neutralized and within thirty minutes she was fine. She went home that night and prepared a tuna casserole in her microwave oven. What do you think happened to her? She had the same severe reaction all over again and went to the hospital emergency room for treatment. But do you think they were able to treat her? No, because they could not figure out what her problem was. It was mercury toxicity! At a later date, the casserole was tested with a vapor tester. Just out of the refrigerator the tuna gave no vapor reading at all. After being warmed in the microwave, it caused the meter to peg the top of the scale! Remember the mercury in fish is in the methyl mercury form.

If you do have a reaction to the patch, there is a simple way to neutralize the reaction. Remove the patch. Wash the area with soap and water. Then take 6 gms (about 1½ tsps.) sodium ascorbate (Vitamin C powder) in water. DO NOT TAKE CALCIUM ASCORBATE. Sodium ascorbate will neutralize the reaction in about 20 minutes or less. You should be certain to have some available during the length of time you have the patch on. Because Vitamin C is able to neutralize the reaction, it is best not to take any for a day prior to starting the test. It could invalidate the test. Remember, the purpose of the test is to determine the degree of your sensitivity to mercury.

You should not wear the patch for more than 24 hours. Nor should you continue to wear the patch *during* the 24-hour period if you have an uncomfortable reaction. If you suspect that you are highly mercury toxic and wish to confirm it with the patch test, you may want to have someone with you when it is administered. This in only a precaution and primarily for your comfort. For instance, if you should experience dizziness, driving would not be advised.

All four screening procedures are designed to help you decide if you should have your amalgams removed. They are not diagnostic of mercury toxicity but should be used to indicate the degree of your sensitivity to mercury. If your symptoms are minor, sequential removal with only basic biochemical coverage will be sufficient to help you with your problems. This should cover the majority of Americans. But for those of you who suffer severe problems, this is not sufficient. You should have the full complement of diagnostic testing so that every means possible can be implemented to help you in your recovery.

Knowing your state of health and body chemistry values prior to amalgam removal will enable your doctor to use all biochemical parameters needed *before* beginning amalgam removal. It will also enable him to guide your progress through follow-up testing after the procedure. Sometimes subtle changes are all that are needed to help push a patient toward good health.

The next six sections will describe the testing procedures which we use and which we teach to doctors around the country.

Diagnostic Testing Procedures — Blood Profile

Some of the screening procedures overlap with the diagnostic procedures, and occasionally research tests are brought into the diagnosis of a specific patient. We do have a standard starting point or minimum number of tests that gives us an adequate basis from which a treatment plan can be established. These tests include:

1. Blood serum profile
2. Complete blood count (CBC) with differential and platelet count.
3. Hair analysis for presence of toxic metals
4. Urinary excretion of mercury
5. Electrical readings
6. Health questionnaire

In the mercury toxic patient we select the specific chemistries from those groups that apply directly to mercury toxicity. This does not imply that the other chemistries are not important. They are just not addressed at the initial appointment.

One common denominator that crops up again and again is mercury's attraction to sulfur-containing compounds in our body. This information is very helpful in explaining some reactions, like low energy when the blood tests look great.

Keep in mind that the changes we will be discussing are *potential* changes. They do not all occur in every mercury toxic patient, nor is toxicity related specifically to how many areas are affected. Overall, if you were to evaluate 100 patients, you would see that greater disease problems are more apt to be associated with greater chemical disturbances. But on an individual basis that doesn't always hold true.

Sulfur bonds are like little handles that chemicals can attach to. Oxygen rides on these handles in hemoglobin. It hops on and off with ease. These are very useful bonds (or binding sites as they are often called) because of the ease of the reaction. Sulfur bonding is like your jumping onto a San Francisco cable car. Compare that to some chemical reactions that resemble getting prepared for a space launch.

Glucose, Cholesterol, Triglycerides

The first place we look in blood serum chemistry is the relationship between glucose, cholesterol and triglycerides. If a person is guilty of dietary sinning, most often all three tests will be elevated. If that is the case, we look to nutritional areas. If mercury is working in this area, we will usually see a slight elevation of glucose (blood sugar) and a suppression of cholesterol. These levels are compared to the "optimum levels" sought in balancing body chemistry and are narrower ranges than the "normal" medical ranges. This is discussed in more detail in Chapter V on Nutrition.

Mercury, by interfering with sulfur binding sites, can cause the glucose level to elevate. If insulin is particularly susceptible to mercury, then the glucose levels can get high enough to be considered diabetic. Chromium, manganese, Vitamin C and dietary intake play a big role in diabetes, so mercury is not the major factor. But it can be a contributing factor that doesn't need to be there and that can complicate getting well.

Cholesterol, one measurement of fats in the blood, is discussed fully later. You will read of the importance of cholesterol as the base for building hormones and Vitamin D, of its relationship to energy levels and of the brain's need for it. Advertising has focused on the negative side of it without letting us in on the fact that it is essential for life. Anyway, the majority of the cholesterol in the blood is manufactured by the body. One particular step in this manufacturing process is vulnerable to mercury. When mercury attacks here, the cholesterol level will be lower than dietary and exercise factors would indicate. This potentially upsets manufacture of hormones (like estrogen and testosterone), leaving the body more susceptible to hormonal imbalances.

The glucose-cholesterol complex of mercury toxicity is suggestive but does not seem to play a major diagnostic role at this time. It could lead to discovery of interferences in diseases related to hormone activity, so it is worth observing — especially if the glucose reaches a diabetic level.

Triglyceride level is another measurement of fats in the blood. A variety of things affect triglycerides. Dietary sinning elevates triglycerides faster than sugar affects glucose. We have seen cases where glucose and cholesterol are in the proper range while the triglyceride level is elevated 100 to 300 points. In some of these cases, triglyceride has dropped 200 points in three days after amalgam removal. In other cases, stress — the type where a person is strapped into an apparently unsolvable problem — will cause several hundred points of elevation. Here's where the doctor has to balance nutrition against emotional stress against mercury. When mercury is the problem with triglyceride, though, changes are dramatic and fast.

Serum Proteins

Blood serum proteins are the next area of interest. Now we are getting down to more specific diagnosis. There are two basic serum proteins. Albumin and globulin. They are active in what is called our immune system. White blood cells and serum proteins are considered together when our body's immune system — or defense system — is discussed.

Many people have heard the term gamma globulin or have even had a gamma globulin shot to bolster their immune system. This is the sort of thing we are discussing. When mercury appears in the blood stream, the immune system will react against it. How does mercury get into the blood stream? Simple.

As mercury vapor comes off the filling, it can be inhaled and can pass from the lungs directly into the blood stream. If it is mixed with food during chewing, it can be swallowed, can go down the digestive tract and be absorbed into the bloodstream.

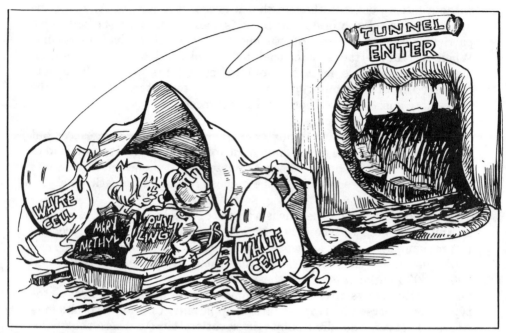

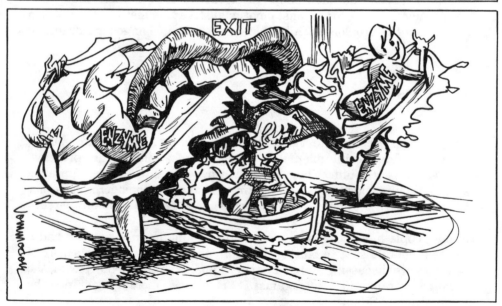

WHITE CELLS AND STRIPPERS IN ACTION

Either way, when it gets there it is going to react. Mercury in vapor form is highly reactive chemically and starts looking for those delicious sulfur bonds. Albumin has some of these tasty sulfurs, so it becomes a favorite dining place for mercury. The mercury grabs hold. When mercury grabs one of these sulfur binding sites, it holds on with a death grip. The globulin usually tries to destroy strangers in the blood. A mercury-albumin compound is definitely a stranger.

Jess Clifford, the giant who came to our aid in the current Amalgam War, is a scientist who knows a lot about the immune system. He has worked out an explanation of what goes on when the body tries to fight a mercury compound. Mercury compounds are not normal "game" for the immune system hunters. They don't know whether to use a cannon, a rifle or a shotgun. (Perhaps over-simplified!) In this quandary, the immune system chooses to cover the mercury compound with a coat of globulin. With a covering of globulin, the compound becomes — in the vernacular — *transparent to the immune system.* In other words, it has become invisible. The immune system no longer includes that compound in its census of strangers.

Looking at the situation from outside the body, the mercury is still floating around in the blood even though it is in a compound covered with globulin. A blood test will show a slightly elevated globulin level. As more mercury seeps into the blood, more coatings appear and the globulin level goes up a little more. Since most people have amalgam in their mouths, this creeping up of the globulin level appears to be a "normal" occurrence and little attention is paid to it.

Since part of the treatment of the mercury toxic patient is to remove this globulin (the process is called globulin stripping), the status of the immune system becomes more and more significant. Observations have suggested to us that a patient's ability to respond after amalgam removal is somehow related to the strength of the immune system. When this idea first began to take form in our minds, we looked at Total Protein levels, albumin levels, globulin levels and the A/G ratio. None of these told us consistently what we needed to find out. Then one day, when we were at 39,000 feet in an airplane, an idea came. Globulin was telling us the story, but only as it was related to the total amount of protein in the blood. We picked a new ratio. The total-protein-to-globulin ratio (TP/G). This is determined by dividing the total protein value by the globulin value. For instance, if the total protein is 7.0 gm% and the globulin is 2.4 gm%, then the TP/G ratio is 2.9.

In looking back over patient records, we found that this ratio did hold a key to diagnosis. Those patients with ratios around 2.9 to 3.1 responded quickly. Those with a ratio below 2.6 responded more slowly and those below 2.1 were in real trouble. How can you change the ratio? We found that Vitamin A and a combination of minerals and digestive enzymes will correct it in most people. The Vitamin A seems to be the biggest single factor though in speeding up recovery reactions.

Now the TP/G ratio is inspected early in diagnosis. Ratios close to 3.0 suggest that we tell the patient to look for a speedy recovery. Lower ratios suggest that the patient pay close attention to dietary intake and watch carefully for other mercury responses that might hamper progress.

Diagnostic Testing Procedures — Hair Analysis

Triad: Calcium, Manganese, Mercury

Hair analysis is the next area to be scrutinized for mercury toxicity. To be a mercury toxic patient, one must first have a problem in what is called the "triad". Imbalance is what is noted. Levels can be either high or low, but *not* close to the optimum level.

Most often calcium is high — especially in the female. Males don't get as high a level of calcium as females do for some unknown reason. High is noted at about 1100 parts per million (ppm) and may go up to 5000 or more in a female. Levels of 2000 ppm are high for a male. At the other end of the scale, it can appear in the 200 to 300 ppm range. In a study of thirty women with PMS (premenstrual syndrome), we found that nearly every one had an elevated calcium level as well as having the general pattern for the mercury toxic patient in other chemistries. Is it possible that such a widespread problem could be caused by amalgams? Remember the interference with hormones that has already been discussed, and add to that the excess calcium levels. It certainly does appear that amalgams could play a very large role in this common female affliction.

There are different interpretations of the various combinations of imbalances in the triad, but let's start with the worst. High calcium-low manganese-low mercury. This combination is seen in the most severe cases and is the toughest to correct. What appears to happen is that mercury combines with a chemical on the cell membrane. (Each cell has its own "skin" and this is termed the cell membrane.) This mercury-chemical combination has an affinity for calcium. When they all get stuck together it appears that oxygen transfer into the cell and carbon dioxide transfer out of the cell runs at lowered efficiency. Clinical observations suggest that mercury is not excreted as effectively when the calcium levels are high and are presumably interfering with mercury transport also.

Manganese is a problem because it seems to be a large factor in all the diseases that have been mentioned. In our studies we have noted that manganese deficiency is apt to be the primary one in all degenerative diseases. Mercury can be toxic in itself. It can form methyl mercury, which is more toxic. And it can inhibit the action of manganese. If manganese acts as a key to unlocking the energy in a cell, and if mercury takes up its position, then the cell doesn't function. The academic question then becomes, does mercury cause the problem or does the lack of manganese cause the problem?

A high manganese produces the same effect as a low manganese because as mineral levels go up beyond the optimum ranges, they appear to be in a nonbiological (inactive) form. They behave as if they are not reactive. This produces the same effect on the body as a low level.

High manganese levels are not common. They are seen roughly 15 percent of the time. Adding a supplement called TransMix helps to rid the body of the inactive material and then fresh minerals can do their work.

Mercury in hair analysis gives us a clue as to what the cells are doing. A low level indicates a lack of ability to excrete, thus we see retention toxicity. High levels indicate a more than average exposure. In the past we thought that low levels suggested low exposure, but that does not seem to be the case. Today low levels suggest that we are going to have difficulty in treating a case. More attention is paid to diet, exercise and other not-so-significant minerals.

Zinc, Potassium

Establishment of the triad (calcium, manganese, mercury) gives a starting point for mercury toxicity as far as hair analysis is concerned. Next we look to two other minerals. If a patient is really toxic, we see the triad extend to zinc and to potassium. Potassium becomes involved in the cases of severe neurological problems — emotional problems, epilepsy, MS.

As a general rule, the more deficient the zinc and potassium (in that order), the more problems the patient is likely to have. They both affect cell membrane permeability, so this could be the core of their action. Both are involved in so many chemical reactions in the body, that it is difficult to pinpoint why they are so important.

Both zinc and potassium can be found in the inactive, excessively high ranges. As in the case with manganese, the symptoms are those of deficiencies. This happens perhaps 5 percent of the time, so it is not a widespread problem. Usually excessive zinc levels are related to eating too much hard cheese. Here hard cheese must be severely restricted for three to six months while the zinc level is optimizing.

There are other minerals that can affect the activity of these five minerals, but they are not dealt with in this book. While we do include them in the diagnosis of mercury toxicity and nutritional deficiencies in patients who come to our office, they are not typical reactors like these five.

Diagnostic Testing Procedures — Complete Blood Count (CBC)

The complete blood count (CBC) is an action-packed analysis. It is the least costly ($10 or less in most areas), yet provides a lot of information for diagnosis and for follow up. We look first at the white cell count. Mercury is toxic, therefore every patient's white cell count will react to placement of amalgams. Mercury is toxic. Most people respond by an increase in their white cells of 2000-3000, but some may go up to 5000-10,000. We have noticed that people without mercury amalgams have white cell counts around 5000 to 5500. Those with amalgam have closer to 7500. Dr. Pinto had said back in 1973 that he and his parents removed amalgams on anyone with a white count consistently above 10,000. After eleven years of watching white cells, we are uncomfortable with anything above 7500.

When white cells are elevated at all, it is well to look at what is called the "differential". This is a count of white cells that divides them into several families. We are finding that some of the families which were thought to be normal for most people do not show up when mercury is not present. These changes can take place in two or three days, which is dramatic when you consider the enormous number of blood cells the body contains.

Overall, the most useful analysis we use parallels one of our most practical discoveries. Most people who suffer from mercury toxicity are constantly fatigued. They sleep more than eight hours a night and wake up tired. Many have been to a physician for "chronic fatigue" and have had a blood test done. The red cells and hemoglobin were excellent so they were told to see a psychiatrist. It's all in their heads!

Well over half of our patients have followed this pattern. They feel insulted by the suggestion that they are using fatigue as a sham to avoid obligation. After seeing this pattern in hundreds of patients, even before we were aware of mercury toxicity, we began to wonder what biochemical explanation could lie behind the "syndrome". Dr. Al Belian, a Detroit dentist who bugs us by dropping new ideas on us every few months, called with an idea that became what we feel is the answer. Remember those sulfur bonds we mentioned in the blood profile section? Al told us that hemoglobin has two of these binding sites on each molecule, and that mercury can easily attach to them.

Then we started thinking. What if???? What if one mercury atom got onto one sulfur position out of the two possible? That hemoglogin's oxygen-carrying capacity would drop 50 percent. Could a 50 percent drop in oxygen make someone feel fatigued? Maybe we had discovered a new kind of anemia. Couldn't inefficient transport produce the same effect as low hemoglobin? Then we noticed another interesting point. Some of these patients had quite good hemoglobin levels — even higher than high normal. And another thing. They had high hematocrits.

Hematocrit used to be called cell volume. That was a good term because it described precisely what your're looking for. Hematocrit is the term used to indicate the percentage of blood that is composed of cells. We have noted that when all biochemical and nutritional systems are balanced, the hematocrit is usually 45-46 percent. "Normal" can extend down to 38 percent. Some of our fatigued patients were running 52-54 percent. That doesn't make sense. Unless . . . suppose the body recognizes that it is not transporting enough oxygen. Suppose it compensates for this by crowding more red blood cells into the blood stream. That would produce a high concentration of low-efficiency hemoglobin. Result? A good looking chemistry and a fatigued, "anemic" patient making the pilgrimage from doctor to doctor.

Another factor from an entirely different area cropped up about the same time. Dr. Olympio Pinto had recorded on videotape the changes in live red blood cells caused by eating pork, smoking cigarettes, drinking caffeine and other similar destructive habits. Of particular interest to us was the profound reaction an hour after a patient ate pork. We noted that more than half of the red blood cells were what are termed "ghosts". Ghosts are red cells that have lost their hemoglobin. This could explain the sleepiness after eating. Most people call it hypoglycemia, but looking at the "live" dead cells, it looks like a lack of oxygen transport is a more logical answer.

Pinto pointed out that amalgam placement does the same thing to red cells. He also suggested that eating could generate enough mercury vapor to "ghost" a significant number of red cells. We asked our pathologist, Dr. David Bowerman, about the situation.

"There were at least 50 percent of the red cells that were non-functional. A red cell is supposed to live 120 days, isn't it? How can you lose half of them and survive?

"The body can regenerate half of its red cells in two days if it has to. But if it does, you will see an elevated alkaline phosphatase and elevated LDH." (These are blood profile tests.)

Finally things began to fit together. Dr. Bowerman's comments on the enzymes applied back to our oxygen-deficient anemia theory. Pulling all the bits of information together, this is what we had. If mercury attaches to hemoglobin binding sites and produces lower oxygen transport, and if low oxygen tension produces a compensatory increase in red cell concentration, and if the body rapidly replaces these contaminated red cells, then the blood will show elevated enzyme levels. We looked at patient chemistries before and after amalgam removal and saw this exact pattern emerge.

In acutely fatigued patients where the bone marrow is still working well, we find elevated hemoglobin and hematocrit levels. Alkaline phosphatase and LDH enzymes in the blood are elevated to the high normal range. Energy is low. After amalgam removal the hemoglobin, hematocrit and both enzymes drop while the energy level climbs.

Now we look at these fatigued patients with high hemoglobin and are quick to tell them that it is *not* all in their heads.

Long-term fatigue is characterized by lower levels of hemoglobin and hematocrit, but they can still fall within the "low normal" range. This is because heavy metals such as mercury interfere with the production of the hemoglobin molecule itself. It interferes with the production of a substance called coenzyme A which is necessary for the formation of not only hemoglobin, but cholesterol as well.

Imagine this problem in combination with the fact that mercury is cutting the efficiency of the hemoglobin which *is* there, and it is easy to see why the patient feels fatigued. *These* levels usually move upward upon amalgam removal. Energy is restored over a period of a few weeks as compared to a few days in the patient with short-term fatigue.

Diagnostic Testing Procedures — Urinary Mercury Excretion

One of our best indicators of toxicity had a stormy development over the past three years. When we started reading American articles on urinary excretion of mercury, the one thing we found consistent was inconsistency. Most of the medical and dental articles we read suggested that high levels of urinary mercury indicated toxicity and conversely low levels indicated health. However . . . almost every article contained a "however" clause such as:

"However, we have seen people with high urinary mercury levels who were apparently in good health and low levels in people who were sick."

None of these statements gave us confidence in their conclusions.

What did the foreign literature show? Dr. Alfred Stock of Germany and Trachktenberg of Russia both felt that they could find toxicity at 1-5 mcg/L (micrograms mercury per liter urine). Rutherford and Johnson said 25 mcg, and Fuhner said 100 mcg. We asked the pathologist at a toxicolgy laboratory, and he said 20 mcg was their red flag level. They would consider 40 mcg as definite toxicity. Looking at the dental literature was like listening to an auction. Dr. Wilmer Eames published a figure of 150 mcg as toxic in a 1971 ADA Journal. In 1981, Dr. P.L. Fan of the American Dental Association established 500 mcg as the upper safe limit. Eames published again in 1983, but did not overbid Fan. He stayed at 500 mcg. Again, we took our dilemma to pathologist Dr. David Bowerman.

"Why don't you call CDC?" he suggested.

That sounded like pretty good advice. CDC is the Centers for Disease Control in Atlanta, Georgia. Any laboratory that does interstate testing has to pass rigorous standards set up by CDC. When an epidemic hits, CDC is our primary defense. When Legionnaire's Disease hit, CDC was called immediately. Sure. It was the logical call to make.

We contacted a toxicologist at CDC and asked who has the ultimate responsibility for setting the standards of safety and toxicity in the U.S.

"We do," was his reply.

"At what level is mercury in urine considered reflective of toxicity?"

"Thirty micrograms per liter."

We asked if dentistry was within CDC jurisdiction. We were told that dentristry is a self-policing organization with high ethical standards and as such is not directly responsible to CDC. He said that dentistry is ultimately responsible to itself.

We then told him of the floating 150 to 500 mcg safety limit that was being advertised by dentistry. He was rather attentive. We asked for a quotable comment, which he readily gave.

"It looks to me like an accommodation for sloppy procedures."

We decided to start testing urine samples for mercury and see what effect — if any — that amalgam removal procedures would have. A really happy accident occurred. Otherwise we might have lost interest in the muddle of information we had collected. Our first patient showed 12 mcg. We tested her again and got a reading of 10 mcg. After amalgam removal her level shot up to 136 mcg, her symptoms improved, her white blood cell count dropped from an average of 17,000 to 10,500 and her body temperature (which had long been subnormal) came up to 98.6 degrees F. Wow! All that in just one day!

That started a long process of watching urine mercury levels. We now consider it one of our most valuable diagnostic tests. We even have a mini-screening program based solely on urinary excretion. It doesn't reveal *everything*, but it does give a good idea of a patient's exposure-excretion condition.

After several years of monitoring urine mercury, today we consider 4-8 mcg in the urine reflective of ridding the body of routine daily exposures from air, food and water. Levels below that suggest either no mercury exposure (rare on this planet) or the inability to excrete mercury.

Patients with the most severe symptoms seem to fall into the category of lower than 4 mcg of excretion. We rarely get these patients to make quantum leaps like our first patient did. But we do note that at these low levels a patient will start feeling perceptible progress when the excretion goes up 100 percent. A person with 1 mcg would have to increase to 2 mcg. Two would have to progress to 4 mcg. After 4 mcg, the percentage is not as important, but it certainly is important in the very low range.

After watching patient progress via urine mercury, we coined the term that we now use of *retention toxicity* to describe the patient who is mercury toxic because of lack of ability to excrete. When the original blueprint of man was drawn there was mercury on the planet. Man probably had the ability to excrete it then and does today. Our observations suggest that the mercury toxic patient loses some of his ability to excrete mercury when amalgam is placed in his mouth. That assumption is based on observing so many patients who had very little in the line of health problems until amalgam was placed. Upon removal of the amalgam, they excreted more mercury and their symptoms abated. In a few of these patients some improvements were noted after half of their amalgams were removed. But most have to have the last fleck removed before they start improving.

We saw this dramatically illustrated in one patient who will be described in detail later. In her case, as each filling was removed she had a series of quite noticeable reactions. Perhaps her reactions to the removal of each filling occurred because she was at that time a universal reactor. Whatever the cause, she certainly gave us an education that day! But then this is not unusual. Every patient we see teaches us something to help other patients.

After amalgam removal, the problem of *retention toxicity* can be confronted without its primary obstacle. If. . .If. . .If. . .If the fillings are removed sequentially. If not, it is really tough to correct retention toxicity.

That brings up the next major diagnostic procedure. It is actually the most important single test, because if it is done properly, success is in sight. If it is violated, failure is assured 90 percent of the time.

Diagnostic Testing Procedures — Electrical Current

If someone were to pin us down as to the mechanism behind the success of sequential removal of amalgam, we would have to say, "We don't know." Observations certainly tell us whether our patient is better or not. But the reason is hidden down in the electrical mechanism of the body. We strongly suspect that the electrical aspects of acupuncture are involved.

As discussed in screening procedures, electrical current is generated in metallic fillings in the mouth. The higher the electrical current, the faster the chemical reactions are taking place. Subsequently, more mercury comes out of the fillings. A more in depth explanation of the mechanism of electrical current is given in the manuscript presented to NIDR as seen in appendix D. If you are interested in more detail, you might like to read that part next.

We knew that electrical current was generated by fillings. That finding was published in 1880 by Patrick. From Pinto's 1976 publication, we learned that in 1940, Lain, Schriever and Caughron wrote that there is almost unanimous agreement that:

"1. The human saliva constitutes a good electrolyte.

2. In every oral cavity containing dissimilar metals all the elements of galvanic cells are present, and

3. That certain symptoms and pathologic lesions in the mouth diagnosed as electrogalvanic lesions disappear after complete and direct replacement with certain metals."

Schoonover and Sounder in 1941 investigated the rate of corrosion of dental amalgam under various conditions and state:

"One has only to examine the surface and base of any dental fillings to observe corrosion, which is probably the result of galvanic action. Such amalgams need not be in contact with other metal or in mouths containing additional metal fillings.

"Galvanic action on a single metal filling may also result from exposure of different areas of the filling to solutions that are not chemically the same. Such a condition produces a simple concentration cell, which in dental practice would be found where an amalgam restoration fails to seal the cavity. The base of such an amalgam would be exposed to a solution of a different concentration, for example of oxygen, from that in contact with the surface."

What we didn't know at that time was how much current was generated, nor did we know whether it held any significance or not.

We bought an electrical meter in 1979 and started touching fillings. After a year of touching the two probes to right and left sides, upper and lower, crisscross and everything we could think of, we had a man come into the office with an oscilloscope to see what we were measuring. As fate would have it, the patient we were testing had both positive and negative electrical current in his fillings.

"What does negative current mean?" asked the man with the oscilloscope.

"How should we know?" The meter we had used didn't say anything about negative fillings.

Well, a lot has happened since that day and we know what negative electrical current means now. It means *bad*. We now even know why. Clincical observation soon taught us that most people with severe cases of multiple sclerosis, epilepsy or emotional disease had lots of negative current fillings. They usually had six or more. About 15 percent had less than six negative fillings and about 5 percent had no negatives. But the trend showed through.

Recently we have found that *Streptococcus mutans* (mentioned earlier) can methylate mercury in the mouth. Methyl mercury is the mercury compound that is so devastating. The chemistry of other methylating bacteria suggests that the environment created immediately over a negative current filling may be conducive to high amounts of methyl mercury formation. Since methyl mercury is 100 times more neurotoxic than elemental mercury, this may explain why some fillings are so detrimental to some people and not to others.

This quizzical finding on electrical current is the difference between success and failure. If the negative fillings are removed first, the patient's chances of improving are good. If the positively charged fillings are removed first — leaving negative behind — chances for success drop to 10 percent or less. The dentist does not have to jump around all over the mouth chasing current. We have found that if all of the fillings are removed from the *quadrant* (¼ of the mouth) with the highest negative readings first, the patient will have an 80 percent chance of getting well. After all the quadrants with negative fillings are completed, then those with high positive current are removed. Following this sequence (called sequential amalgam removal) has proven to be a very effective way of removing fillings. We still have a number of patients who heard about mercury toxicity, ran out and had their fillings removed at random and have yet to show any improvement.

Looking back at the 70s now, we know why our patients only responded 10 percent of the time. We always removed fillings by starting in the upper left quadrant. Why? Just because that's where we *always* started. No science — just a habit. Possibly about one time in ten we coordinated with coincidence and treated a patient whose highest negative current was in the upper left quadrant.

There is still so much we don't know about the electrical current, but we have some good men working with us to find out. The department of electrical engineering at one of our American Universities is trying to springboard from a European University study on what the biological significance of this electrical current might be, but so far they are runn-

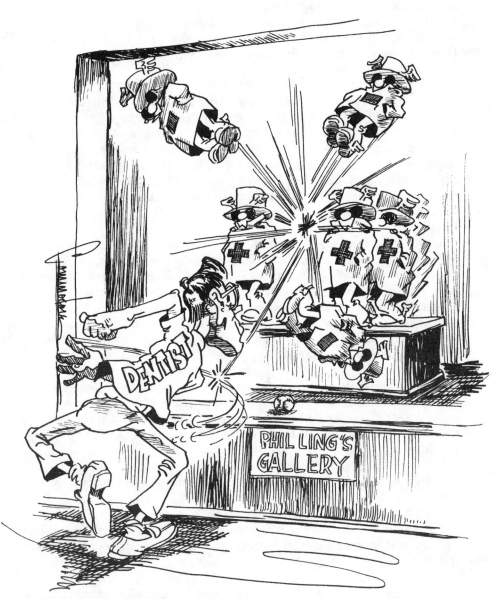

FROM A NEGATIVE "PHIL LING"...TO A POSITIVE ONE

ing into complex blind alleys. Electrical current is generated on the surface of single fillings, between two fillings that touch and between the filling and the dentinal fluid beneath the filling. That makes for complexity. They have suggested that changes in heart function may be related to brain current changes and not from direct effects from the fillings to the heart muscle. There is so much unknown at this time that they don't even want their name mentioned until they have a better handle on explanations. Our personal thanks to J.F. for his hours of searching and frustration. We wish you Godspeed.

Back to the practical side of electrical current for just a minute. What does it mean if you touch the tooth with the probe of the Amalgameter (the instrument we use to measure the current) and the meter doesn't show a reading — negative or positive? This means that the filling is either pure gold (gold foils usually do not register current), that it is a composite (which usually doesn't have a current unless Dycal is used as a base) or that it is an amalgam which is highly corroded.

When a filling has undergone heavy corrosion, there is a layer of corrosion on the outer surface. Often the probe cannot get through this layer even when the filling is scratched. If this is the case, we recommend that a dental bur be used to polish the filling so that the probe can get past the corrosion layer. In about 80 percent of the cases we find these fillings to be negative. Is it possible that negative current, in addition to being related to higher production of methyl mercury, is also related to higher corrosion rates? What type of relationship really exists here?

In Chapter VII we will discuss dental materials in greater detail, but there are a few things to remember which we consider to be extremely important. The first is that gold and amalgam should not be in the mouth at the same time. If you are having your amalgams replaced with gold, all amalgam should be removed first and then the gold crowns placed. You can have plastic temporary crowns placed until all the amalgam has been removed. Under no circumstances would we now put gold in the same mouth which contains amalgam. This increases the amount of electrical current tremendously and can lead to severe heart or allergy problems in those who are susceptible to these diseases.

What do we consider high current? Voll of Germany recommends against the presence of more than 6 microamps of current. He suggests that greater amounts of current affect the acupuncture meridians in the body adversely and contribute to disease processes. You can think of these meridians as violin strings running from the top of the body through the teeth and to the bottom of the feet. We become concerned about *negative* current at 1 microamp. We feel that some of the dramatic improvements we have seen in some of our patients are due to changes in their electrical field as a result of removing negative fillings in addition to getting rid of the mercury.

Gold crowns can have very high electrical currents, but they are seldom negative. If the gold alloy (crowns are not made of pure gold because it is too soft) contains palladium, the current can be quite high. We usually do not recommend that these be removed unless you still have symptoms that have not cleared up after all amalgam has been out of the mouth for a few weeks. Under *no* circumstances do we recommend the new non-precious (nickel) crowns. Many of these crowns exhibit negative current and it is usually quite high.

The last thing we would like to note about electrical current and treatment is that in the case of the suicidal patient, if there is very much negative current, it may be wise not to remove all of the amalgam in one quadrant at the same time. The suicidal patient is extremely friable in terms of reaction to electrical change. We strongly recommend that the suicidal patient be given PZI (protamine zinc insulin) in the area of the amalgam removal at each appointment and that this patient have some-one with him at all times for the first 24 hours after the procedure.

As you can see from reading this section, electrical current is a very important aspect of treatment for mercury toxicity. We hope soon to understand more about the *why* of electrical current. But in the mean-time we again want to caution you against having your fillings removed in random order. Sequential amalgam removal is a must for the patient with multiple or severe symptoms.

While we've discussed electrical current at great length in this section, there is another factor of equal importance to the success of treatment. This second factor is supplementation with nutrients which encourage the cell membrane to allow stored mercury to be excreted. This biochemical coverage must be started prior to initial amalgam removal. A more thorough discussion of supplementation is found in chapter V.

Diagnostic Testing Procedures — Questionnaire

Questionnaires are interesting tests. They give information on the patient's current status, but more than that, they can educate an observer. We're not sure where the education is headed, but we are noticing trends in symptoms. We have noted, for instance, that people with numbness and tingling in their fingers and toes have low manganese levels. Given long enough they can end up with multiple sclerosis.

If they have numbness and MS, they eventually can have heart irregularities and emotional problems. From there they can proceed to fatigue and a series of hormonal disturbances possibly related to sulfur interference.

If this information could be combined with patient chemistries, we might find ways to push that 80 percent success rate even higher. We hope to have a program soon to be able to put this type of data on our computer.

The analyses discussed in this chapter — blood, hair, CBC, urine mercury, electrical current — plus the questionnaire as seen for each patient give sufficient data to allow a trained clinician to diagnose and plan treatment for the average mercury toxic patient. Really, a lot can be done for even severe cases of epilepsy, arthritis, allergies and the other diseases mentioned throughout the book. But there is always more. Perfection is always elusive. There are unending numbers of frontiers to explore.

Research Testing Procedures of Interest

We have taken a peek into some of these new frontiers. It would be nice to test all the frontier parameters on every patient, but cost and lack of training in interpretation make us hesitant.

On the chance that you might like to share our peek into potential future research, here are our observations.

Cell Morphology Under Hoffman Optics

The most exciting area of current research, and the one with the greatest potential, is cell morphology as seen under Hoffman Optics. *Morphology* refers to the size and shape of cells and their internal structures. Cell morphology is the study of changes within a red or white blood cell as a result of a challenge to the immune system. The study of cell morphology has the potential to be the single most accurate method of determining toxicity or biocompatibility. Hoffman Optics is a type of microscope system that allows you to see great detail in a red or white cell in a three dimensional mode. Conventional "bright field" microscopes tend to burn out small parts of the cells visually so you can't see detail as well. The problem is that only a handful of people in America know how to identify and interpret these morphologic changes.

We have seen hundreds of slides of cells under the direction of Jess Clifford. Jess understands human health-disease problems as reflected in white cells better than any person around. He can point out changes in the nuclear membrane within a white cell that occur when a person has a cancerous tumor. If surgery is performed and the tumor is totally removed, the little whip-like appendages disappear. What really concerns us is that when an amalgam is placed, those little whips appear in just the same manner. Amalgam removal produces the same type of reduction in them. To our untrained eyes, these whips are easy to see. We would suggest that they could become an indicator of toxicity. To test a new material for biocompatability, look at the cells, then place the material and look again. In three to four days significant changes occur, so you don't have to wait for months or sacrifice an animal to tell whether the test material passes this test or not.

Another thing of interest that we have been taught by Jess is the twenty-one day cycle of the immune system. The easiest way to describe what this means is to say that approximately 21 days after a challenge to the immune system, it decides to take a vacation. If an immune challenge occurs on Day #1 and a second one occurs on Day #21 while the immune system is on vacation, the patient is highly susceptible to severe disease. Is this perhaps why some people with amalgam have diseases and others don't? We think it could play a part in the entire process. The immune challenges that we have isolated thus far as being associated with MS are the flu, a cold and cholera shots. Should these things happen 21 days before or after an amalgam is placed, you are set up for problems. Do you always know what you will be doing in 21 days? If you do, then go ahead and have amalgam or nickel placed. But if you can't tell what the future holds for you 21 days down the road, we advise that you never have amalgams or nickel placed again. It is also better that you not have your dental appointments to remove your amalgam all on the *same* day of the week. By the third appointment you have hit that 21st day. Vary your appointment day so that you do not challenge your immune system with the amalgam removal either.

Electroencephalogram

We have heard from people who develop devices that measure brain waves that aluminum temporary crowns can change the brain's alpha waves up to 1000 percent. That sounds impressive, but we're not sure what an alpha wave is.

We have reports that electroencephalograms in seizure patients were "abnormal" before amalgam removal and "normal" afterward. How?

How much? In what area? "Dentists" aren't allowed to have that information. Some day we'll have a "real doctor" on our staff and we can find out their secrets. Might they be helpful? Our philosophy is "You never know until you look."

Psychological Testing

"People process thought differently with amalgams than they do after amalgam removal. They cope better."

That's what we have to go on from a psychologist's report. Perhaps we need a standardized test instead of the one we have (only the designer has the key). We have waited a long time and have money invested in this testing but no useful information has been given us by the psychologist so far. From what we see happening to our depressed and suicidal patients, we know something is happening. What? It looks as if we'll have to wait *another* year to find out. We don't mind developing patience, but we want it now!

Jaro Pleva (1983) in relating his experiences when physicians were unable to help him with his complaints and health problems said,

> "The diagnosis that all this was because of stress or strained relations in the family I could not take seriously. From my previous life I was used to more stress, both psychic and physical than during this period.
>
> About five months after the last amalgam filling had been removed some relatively strong symptoms returned for a period of one to two weeks . . . After this period I had a feeling of even better well-being than before.
>
> The improvements in my health could not be related to any factor in my surroundings . . . Finally I want to stress the amazing improvement in well-being, only three months after the final dental treatment. In spite of still improving, I have regained a feeling of peace and calmness, of being able to appreciate smells, details and graduations in my surroundings, something I must go back 10-15 years to find."

In his list of symptoms in his article he described his emotional and psychological problems as being those of severe amnesia, constant strain, anxiety, irritability, difficulty and even impossibility to control behaviour, indecision, loss of interest in life, tiredness and a feeling of being old.

Body Temperature

Mercury toxic patients frequently have low body temperatures. Why? It could be mercury blocking thyroid activity. Thyroid has four little binding sites. Sound familiar? Sulfur binding sites! What happens if mercury gets on one of those sites? The blood test for thyroid might *look* good, but is the function the same?

Usually within 24 hours of final amalgam removal, body temperature has sought 98.6 degrees F. It may not make it all the way, but even 96's and 97's can get at least into the 98 degree category. There is bound to be a hormonal problem involved, but which one? How much? Does dentistry have the right to place something in your mouth that lowers your body temperature 1 or 2 degrees? Is it really significant? Whose body is it?

Fundus Photography Of The Retina

The eyes have it. What do they have? Mercury. Doty Murphy, MD called several years ago asking if we had an ophthalmoscope. That is an instrument to look at the retina in the back of the eyeball. We didn't have one, but the fellow next door did. When we looked through it, all we could positively identify was our eyelash.

Doty described black streaks that occur in the retina. Professionally they are considered to be areas where the elongated near-sighted eye has put tension on the retina and stretched it so that we see underlying epithelium below the retina showing through. Dr. Murphy had noted that these occurred in people who had amalgams and were absent in people without amalgam. Another strange event is that when amalgams are removed, the black areas begin to disappear. We now have some progress photographs to demonstrate this.

Dentists see black spots, too. In the mouth they are called amalgam tatoos. Origin? Yes, there is a very logical explanation. The dentist (the sloppy one across the street, not yours) slipped with the drill and cut up the gums slightly. Then when he placed the amalgam, he inadvertently pressed some of it into the cut tissue and didn't wash it out. What you see is the amalgam "tatooed" into the tissues.

That explanation satisfied us until we found amalgam tatoos in the roof of the mouth, down the bony ridge an inch away from a lower tooth and finally — the one that did it — one on the uvula. The uvula is that little finger-like projection at the very back of your soft palate. Convince us that a dentist hit that with a drill and then smeared amalgam into it! There aren't enough sloppy dentists to account for the number of amalgam tatoos we see.

Do you suppose those dark areas in the retina are amalgam tatoos? Do they affect vision? Some people think they do. Ask around. When did you start wearing glasses for nearsightedness? When did you get your first amalgams? Was it within six months? Some optometrists feel that myopia (near sightedness) and cataracts are related to mercury in fish and amalgam. Research is going on in these areas as well.

Yes, all of these are new frontiers. They can all potentially tell us a lot about the ways in which mercury and other heavy metals can affect us biologically. We would encourage our scientists and university professors to begin earnest work in as many of these areas as possible.

CHAPTER V

Nutrition's Vital Role In
Recovery From Mercury Toxicity

Supplementation

Having detected evidence of mercury poisoning, measured its biological effects through diagnostic blood chemistry procedures, and eliminated the source of the poison by *sequential* amalgam removal, there remains the crucial task of getting rid of the body's stored mercury. This step offers an exciting chance for our patients to take an *active* role in their recovery.

Good nutrition improves the body's ability to perform oxygen exhange and toxin elimination. Poor nutrition inhibits exchange of oxygen and slows elimination of toxins. When the body has undergone the stress of prolonged exposure to a toxin like mercury, we cannot take the months or years required to rebuild through diet alone. This is when supplementation is required. To us, nutrition is defined as proper supplementation plus good foods when both are matched to your body's needs.

In 16 years of monitoring body chemistry and nutrition, we have found that the majority of health conscious people overdose on supplements. We suggest supplementation for many of our patients in our body chemistry practice, but they are primarily based on needs pointed out in blood chemistry and other physiological analyses. Occasionally a supplement is prescribed based on symptoms alone when we have already seen many similar chemistries of people with the same problem.

Supplementation in fact provides an *imbalanced* diet. That may sound strange at first, but consider that a sick person usually has an unbalanced chemistry. Frequently we supply the opposite imbalance to correct it. Many chemistries work on a teeter-totter effect and increasing one will decrease the other one. After the chemistry is fairly stable, maintenance supplmentation can allow us to pick up most of what we need from a good, well-balanced diet.

In supplementing the recovering mercury toxic patient, there is a standard regimen that we use which serves to correct the *basic* chemistry problems. From there, additional supplementation is based on what the patient's chemistry dictates are highs and lows which need correction.

This basic supplementaton regimen serves three primary purposes:

1) to encourage excretion of mercury from the cells by
   a) conditioning the cell membrane
   b) mobilizing mercury from tissue stores
   c) separating mercury from proteins in the blood
      (globulin stripping)
   d) excreting mercury in the urine

2) to help prevent exacerbation of symptoms

and

3) to give the patient a nutrient base for rebuilding damaged tissues

Clinical observations over the past 16 years have shown us that certain combinations of minerals apparently help the cell membrane to become more flexible. If the cell membrane is "sluggish", it has difficulty letting oxygen into the cell and even more difficulty letting mercury out. To increase this exchange we use a tablet called TransMix. It has magnesium, zinc and other minerals that are known to help control cell membrane permeability. The important part is that they are in a certain *ratio* to each other. This helps condition the membranes within 48 hours. For this reason, we recommend that supplementation be started a *minimum* of 48 hours prior to amalgam removal.

The minerals in TransMix are in a highly absorbable form. With five different routes of absorption we can be certain of touching at least one "absorption button" in each patient. Once one of the minerals has been absorbed, regardless of which route worked, the cell becomes more permeable and an even greater absorption rate is achieved.

Mobilizing the mercury is done by a combination tablet called X-IT. It contains selenium, Vitamin E, folic acid and other minerals whose biological activities suffer from interference by mercury. We found it very effective for people who have a great deal of difficulty excreting mercury. In other words — the ones with low urinary mercury excretion. When this combination increased the urinary excretion for the tough cases, we knew it would do well for people with moderate problems. Recent observations indicate that X-IT is so effective at encouraging the release of stored mercury, that this mercury can get backed up in the blood stream.

Mercury in the blood stream is highly reactive and tends to combine with proteins in the blood. Mercurial compounds get coated with globulin as described earlier and cannot be readily excreted. We use a digestive enzyme called Eater's Digest to perform what is termed "globulin stripping". This removes the globulin from the mercurial compound and evidently splits the mercury off the compound. Two Eater's Digest tablets per one X-IT tablet are necessary to accomplish this. Evidence of this is seen when the blood serum globulin level goes down within a few days. Also the Total Protein to Globulin Ratio (TP/G) ratio will move toward its favorable range of 2.9 to 3.1 if everything is going smoothly.

Vitamin C must be standing by to prevent the reactions from "biological reversal" — when the mercury starts dumping into the blood stream. The ascorbate portion of the vitamin C attaches to the mercury to form mercury ascorbate which can then be excreted in the urine.

Vitamin C also helps to rebuild tissues damaged by the toxicity as does TransMix. Both vitamin C and TransMix are good maintenance supplements even after the amalgams are removed. They help replace nutrients burned up in the stress of day-to-day activity.

This regimen — Transmix, X-IT, Eater's Digest and vitamin C — is somewhat standard for the common chemical problems created in the mercury toxic patient. Potassium, zinc and the frequently ultra-disturbed manganese may have to be supplemented in the more severe cases. Where the TP/G ratio is low, vitamin A is effective in raising the ratio and thus giving more impetus to the immune system.

Hormones, especially insulin in the form of PZI (protamine zinc insulin), thyroid and posterior pituitary find their way into the patients' biochemical coverage on occasion. And the age-old standby of activated charcoal has usefulness. It was one of the world's first detoxifiers and is finding new uses in modern science.

After the initial stages of ups and downs that are common during recovery, supplementation usually drops to TransMix, vitamin C and an occasional X-IT. We have all heard older folks say, "It's gonna rain tomorrow. I know because my joints hurt today." There seems to be a scientific basis behind this. When the barometric pressure drops, mercury excretion in the urine slows down and symptoms reappear. X-IT seems to be able to counter that and help keep mercury excretion up. It's nice to keep X-IT on hand for "rainy days."

We have not discussed specific dosages because they are dependent upon each patient's individual chemistry. Supplementation recommendation is part of the well-planned treatment regimen necessary for reversal of problems and should not be abused. Self-medication with everything on the health food store shelf can do more damage than good. Some can actually interfere with cell membrane permeability and prevent mercury excretion.

Nutritional Do's and Don't's For The Mercury Toxic Patient

We have a complete nutritional program available to the patients who come to us for diagnosis of mercury toxicity. The primary purpose of the program is to make you aware of the general things which will affect the speed with which you improve. Many dietary factors adversely affect cell membrane chemistry thus slowing down the ability to excrete toxins. Many of these same factors are an insult to the hormonal balance as well.

The secondary purpose of the program is to enable you to learn about specific foods which have a bad effect upon your body's chemistry. The program isn't designed to "cure" health problems but is designed to complement the treatment regimen for mercury toxicity. It also teaches you what your ideal body chemistry should be and how you can reach that goal if you desire to.

We ask only 85 percent adherence to the entire nutritional program. This is sufficient to accomplish our goals for you and still enables you to have a good mental attitude. Since application of all the principles of the program is not always easy and involves changing many lifelong habits, the decision to stay on the program is not always an easy one. But it is well worth the effort, not only during the period of treatment for mercury toxicity, but for the rest of your life.

We will make reference from time to time to the effect of trace minerals and diet on the endocrine glandular system. Endocrine glands produce hormones: The thyroid gland manufacturers thyroxine hormone; the pancreas produces insulin; adrenalin is a product of the adrenal gland and the sex glands produce testosterone and estrogen. These, plus the hormone output of many more endocrine glands, comprise the regulatory system of the body. Heat production, pulse, blood pressure, sweating and all the normal daily processes of the human body that we are not even aware of are kept in balance by hormones. Minerals help to keep hormones in balance. A deficiency of minerals can result in hormone function lower than optimum. Remember that one of the effects of mercury on the biologic system is interference with hormones. If we are to correct the entire problem, it is necessary to remove as many insults to this system as possible.

We feel that the word "diet" must be defined at this point. For our purposes here it refers *solely* to the *quality* of food eaten and not the amount.

We examine food digestion from two aspects: the blood profile and the mineral analysis of hair. Blood tells us how the body is metabolizing the food we eat and whether nutrients necessary for replacing worn out cells are being adequately provided.

Hair analysis tells us the amounts of minerals that are available within the cells to activate energy-producing molecules. Remember, blood serum is analyzed to learn how food is being broken down and made available to the cells. "Cellular" minerals refer to the metabolism within the cell.

Finally we need to clarify the abstract terms "active" and "inactive". The difference between the two is that active compounds work naturally within the human system while inactive material is not reflected in human biochemical reactions. It occupies space which would be better occupied by active elements and contributes to inefficient body operations.

Though the entire nutritional program goes into more than 17 blood tests and 11 mineral levels, we discuss here only those directly involved with mercury toxicity.

We will look at eight blood tests:

Phosphorus	Glucose
Cholesterol	Triglycerides
Total Protein	Albumin
Alkaline Phosphatase (Alk Phos)	Lactic Dehydrogenase (LDH)

The seven trace minerals to be discussed are:

Calcium	Zinc
Manganese	Potassium
Mercury	Magnesium
	Chromium

Now let's take these one at a time. Please remember, though, that the body is quite dynamic. There are numerous systems working every second and many of these are affected by the same factors.

Endocrine Balance

The relative balance of the endocrine system is reflected by the serum phosphorus level. When it is low, we know there is a hormonal disturbance somewhere, but we don't know exactly what it is. In the days when we were doing only Body Chemistry (nutritional and biochemical counseling), we had to look at several different hormone levels if dietary corrections failed to help. Today, we see quite rapid improvement once amalgam removal has been completed. This assumes that dietary factors are also being addressed at the same time.

Endocrine balance can be illustrated as a teeter-totter with phosphorus on one side by itself and glucose, cholesterol and triglycerides on the other side.

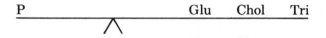

It really looks out of balance doesn't it?

The dietary factors which raise the glucose, cholesterol and triglycerides also cause the depression of the phosphorus. So it is necessary, then, to avoid those foods which cause this elevation. They are primarily sugar, alcohol and caffeine. Any time these items are in the diet there will be an endocrine imbalance. They interfere with the production of hormones by the endocrine glands. As we said before, phosphorus is a reflection of this balance. When it is in the ideal range, the endocrine system is in relative balance. If sugar, alcohol or caffeine pushes up the glucose, cholesterol or triglycerides, then the endocrine function is slowed and the phosphorus is pushed down.

One of the methods we use to help identify the mercury toxic patient is the relationship between glucose and cholesterol. We look first at the glucose level. If it is elevated, we look then to cholesterol. Where dietary infractions are elevating the glucose, the cholesterol will also be elevated. But if the cholesterol is lower than the ideal level while the glucose is elevated, then we suspect mercury interference with the body's ability to form cholesterol.

Glucose

Glucose is a measurement of the blood sugar level. The body converts nearly all the food we eat into glucose because it is necessary for life. But when the glucose remains continuously elevated, many tissues are constantly bathed in it. This is very unhealthy. For example, by use of an instrument called a Periotron, we can demonstrate the amount of glucose in the fluid which surrounds the tooth. Persons with high levels of glucose show greater amounts of periodontal (gum) disease than those with ideal levels. The higher the glucose, the more severe the disease.

Glucose in the body acts to provide adequate energy. If it is maintained at an even, moderate (or as we prefer — ideal) level, the energy level remains constant. The entire body can depend upon a sufficient but not overly abundant supply of glucose. But if something elevates the glucose sharply, then the biological systems are overloaded. At this point, the pancreas detects the elevation and produces insulin to "burn up" the excess glucose. Why? Because the body has been designed to run at an even level known as homeostasis. When this is disturbed, the entire body is affected. We know that clinically we see elevations in glucose levels with the beginnings of degenerative diseases — those which gradually wear the body down rather than those which are caused by bacteria. So we want to see this blood chemistry controlled.

Many things can elevate the glucose level. All drugs — whether prescription or OTC (over-the-counter) — can elevate it. But we are primarily interested here in nutritional influences. Sugar, alcohol, caffeine and fruit juices are the most damaging factors in the diet. Sugar and fruit juices do most of their damage because they are partitioned foods. This means that they have been stripped of the vitamins, minerals and enzymes which enable the body to metabolize or break them down. They are dumped headlong into the glucose metabolic pathway and are very quickly transformed into glucose, thus elevating it and causing the body to have to compensate for it.

This is like racing your car up to 150 mph (that's illegal, isn't it?) and then slamming on the brakes. The more you do this to your car, the sooner it will wear out, right? Having foods and drinks with sugar in them is like running your car up to that excessive speed. Insulin production is the slamming on of the brakes.

Alcohol, caffeine and fruit juices have the same affect on the glucose. We caution all diabetics to avoid not only sugar, but caffeine as well. One cup of coffee can elevate the glucose level enough to need three units of insulin to counteract it.

There are other factors which must be in balance to keep an ideal glucose. Certain minerals are necessary for activation of enzyme systems involved in glucose metabolism. Chromium is known as a part of the Glucose Tolerance Factor. It works at the cell membrane to increase its permeability and enable the glucose to get into the cell instead of remaining in the blood stream or in the fluids around the cell. A deficiency of chromium can be caused by too much refined carbohydrate (sugar, alcohol, white flour, etc.) in the diet.

Zinc is a part of the insulin molecule itself. When zinc is deficient, production of insulin may not be adequate to control glucose in the presence of a high carbohydrate diet. Mercury plays a part in causing zinc deficiency as well as inactivating the insulin molecule.

Manganese also helps to control the glucose level, as does magnesium. Both of these minerals are excreted by the diuretic effect of alcohol and show yet another reason why alcohol causes an increased glucose.

Finally, vitamin C is necessary in the control of glucose. Anything which destroys vitamin C can potentially increase glucose — smoking, stress, drugs, dietary factors, etc.

So what can you do to be certain that you are not nutritionally interfering with the treatment for mercury toxicity in lowering the glucose? Avoid sugar, alcohol, caffeine, fruit juice and refined carbohydrates. Substitutes for these are explained in our diagnostic programs. Eat more protein — turkey, beef — and avoid partitioned and overcooked foods. And, of course, avoiding tobacco products would help as well.

Cholesterol

High levels of cholesterol are caused by sugar, alcohol and caffeine primarily. Recent weight loss, stress, insufficient thyroid function, tobacco, drugs (especially antihistamines) and low mineral levels (chromium, magnesium, calcium and manganese) are other causes. Did you notice that in this whole list we did not list one food that contains cholesterol such as eggs, butter, etc? This is because these things will *not* raise the cholesterol if sugar, alcohol and caffeine are out of the diet and the other factors are eliminated. Sugar raises it perhaps more than anything else and therefore, control of cholesterol is impossible when sugar is in the diet. Many patients on medication to "lower" the cholesterol have completely eliminated their medications by controlling their diet.

Remember the teeter-totter we described earlier? The normal relationship between glucose and cholesterol when sugar, alcohol or caffeine is in the diet is that they are both elevated. But in the mercury toxic patient we usually find the glucose elevated with a deficient cholesterol. Many functions are affected when this is the case. If we do not get cholesterol through dietary intake, the body will produce its own because of the importance of these functions. In fact, 80 percent of all cholesterol in the blood serum is produced by the body from foods which do not contain cholesterol. What functions could be so important? Here are just a few.

One area of interest to nearly everyone who would like to lose weight is that ingested fats enable nutrients to be absorbed. Since *true* hunger is nothing more than the body's search for nutrients, fats help prevent hunger. So weight control is dependent upon the proper fats in the diet — assuming of course that sugar, alcohol and caffeine are *out* of the diet.

Cholesterol is found in the myelinated nerve sheath which is the protective layer that insulates against erratic electrical charges — one of the problems with the MS patient.

Cholesterol is necessary for proper brain function. More than 10 percent of the dry weight of the brain is composed of cholesterol.

Cholesterol is part of the insulation layer around the heart so proper dietary fats help to protect against heart disease.

Cholesterol is necessary for the manufacture and transport of the sex hormones — testosterone and estrogen — so it is important that during puberty youngsters have sufficient butter rather than margarine in order to have proper sexual maturation.

Cholesterol is necessary as a raw material needed in the production of energy in the red blood cells.

One fourth of all of the enzyme systems are dependent upon fats and upon absorption of nutrients through the intestines which is via fat solubility. Therefore all of the enzymes involved in the cell membrane transport system are cholesterol-dependent. This is important because if we do not have proper cell membrane transport (ability to get nutrients into and out of the cells), then we are not getting the benefit of the minerals that we are taking, whether by supplement or in our food.

Cholesterol and vitamin E also help prevent what scientists call "clinkers" from entering the cells. These are chemical compounds which cause cancer and are prevalent in areas of high pollution.

What does all this mean to the mercury toxic patient? It means that you should do everything possible to achieve an ideal level of cholesterol to help you overcome the effects of mercury in all of the areas listed above. Heavy exercise, emotional stress and medications such as aspirin and other salycilates can lower cholesterol levels so these should also be avoided.

On the other hand, we don't want to see an artificially elevated level of cholesterol either. So sugar, alcohol and caffeine should be eliminated (through proper substitutes). When this has been accomplished, two eggs and one quarter lb. butter should be included in the diet daily.

Even before our knowledge of mercury toxicity, we had our patients on this regimen. We found that with sugar, alcohol and caffeine out of the diet and with eggs and butter in the diet, the body would optimize its cholesterol level. Lows were elevated to the ideal level and highs were dropped to the ideal level.

Triglycerides

Triglycerides, like cholesterol, are fats in the blood. They are very large, thick particles which interfere with proper function of the body's chemistry. They cause extra work for the cardiovascular system and should be kept as low as possible.

Like glucose and cholesterol, triglycerides are elevated by sugar, alcohol and caffeine. They are also elevated by stress or by one's perception of stress. We see this test elevated in the mercury toxic patient. Again, getting rid of the amalgam will lower the triglycerides, but the dietary factors must also be under control at the same time if ideal levels are to be reached.

The most important thing you can do as a mercury toxic patient to control the triglycerides level is to avoid sugar, alcohol and caffeine. The next biggest factor in their elevation is smoking, which causes the body to process heavy metals like mercury ineffectively and thus slows down your progress.

Total Protein, Albumin

You've been told about the importance of the Total Protein to Globulin Ratio (TP/G) in determining the ability of your immune system to fight the effects of mercury toxicity. You know now that vitamin A stimulates the immune system. And you know that mercury can "hit" the immune system, rendering it less effective (elevated white cells, decreased lymphs, etc). Now let's look at how you can affect your immune system nutritionally through improper protein metabolism.

The first thing to realize is that there must be sufficient protein in the diet to stimulate the immune system. As is also recommended for those suffering from the condition known as Candidiasis, this must be animal protein. For those of you who are strict vegetarians, we must let you know that your progress will be extremely slow (if you progress at all). We strongly recommend that you discontinue vegetarianism during your treatment period in order to allow the protein fractions in the blood serum to reach a good level. This can be done with eggs and turkey if you prefer to avoid red meats. But we have never seen it happen without any animal protein.

The second thing to realize about protein is that the more it is cooked, the less nutrient it has available for your body's use. Beef should be eaten at least medium-rare and should preferably be grassfed rather than fattened in a feed lot. Wild game like venison is an excellent protein source.

When proteins are completely metabolized, amino acids are produced. These are the building blocks from which new protein is produced to rebuild the body's tisssues. If we interfere with this breakdown process along the way, we produce uric acid instead of amino acids. Our purpose here is to help you do those things which give you an ideal level of globulin and albumin, otherwise known collectively as the Total Protein.

We control protein metabolism chemistries by decreasing liquids with meals to no more than four ounces of liquid during the meal and none for 30 minutes prior to and after the meal. Why are liquids so important in protein metabolism? Go back for a moment to your high school chemistry class. Do you remember that when you studied chemical reactions, you found that anything which diluted the reaction slowed it down? This is true of the breakdown of protein in the stomach. In order to begin the breakdown of protein we must have a sufficient supply of hydrochloric acid (HCl). If we have diluted this acid as well as the other digestive enzymes with liquid prior to or during the meal, then it is no longer strong enough to efficiently initiate the beginning steps of metabolism. Therefore, larger protein particles must go into the steps which come next. Because the initial breakdown is inefficient the whole system suffers. (This is one of the causes of allergies.)

We must make certain that we have sufficient HCl to begin with, and this is where table salt comes into the health picture. The Cl from NaCl (sodium chloride, table salt) is used to produce HCl (hydrochloric acid). Patients on low-salt diets are restricting their ability to metabolize protein. And though it is slightly off the subject at hand, we have never seen an elevated sodium level from table salt. It comes from sodium preservatives such as those found in soft drinks and margarine (sodium benzoate) and in processed foods (sodium nitrates). It also is caused by water softeners, MSG and aspirin. So *if you have sugar, alcohol and caffeine out of your diet,* you do not need to be worried about table salt.

Let's talk just a moment about milk as a problem in protein metabolism. This is a problem for children as well as for adults. Milk is a base which neutralizes acid. As a liquid consumed at meals, it not only dilutes the HCl, but it also neutralizes it. The stomach was designed to be efficient at a very low pH which means a very high acid content. Milk changes this pH so that it is more basic and in this way blocks the absorption of magnesium and calcium in the stomach. This is one of the reasons why milk causes so many allergies. An allergy is a response of the immune system to any "foreign looking" particle. Large protein particles that were not broken down in the stomach properly are such "foreign" objects known as allergens.

Caffeine and alcohol are also both bad about upsetting this balance.

Albumin is the fraction of the Total Protein which enables nutrients to be transported through the blood stream so that they can be made available to the cells. If albumin is low, it does not matter what quality of food you have eaten. There is no more nutrient available from good foods than from poor ones if the albumin is not able to transport them. Again, decreased fluids during mealtime, increased intake of proteins and use of digestive enzymes will help. It also helps to get rid of mercury toxicity which increases globulin levels due to the necessity of the globulin blocking action described in our discussion of the complete blood count.

What then are your primary concerns as a mercury toxic patient with respect to protein metabolism? Avoid liquid in excess of four ounces at mealtime and use digestive enzymes (the one we use is called Eater's Digest) where serum protein metabolism tests are either higher or lower than the ideal level. Eliminate milk, alcohol and caffeine as liquids with meals entirely. Make certain there is enough salt in the diet to allow sufficient hydrochloric acid production. And finally, make certain that your protein is not overcooked. Beef should be eaten as rare as possible. Turkey, of course, should be fully cooked — but not completely cremated. At this time we do not recommend pork or chicken as sources of protein because of their detrimental effect on the blood cells as we saw in Dr. Pinto's video tape. Neither do we recommend salt water fish or shell fish for the mercury toxic patient. They are heavily contaminated with methyl mercury and can slow down the excretion of mercury.

Lactic Dehydrogenase (LDH), Alkaline Phosphatase (Alk Phos)

LDH and Alk Phos are liver enzymes. Liver function is the last line of defense. If the liver malfunctions, amino acids and vitamin levels in the body drop because they aren't being synthesized. Both LDH and Alk Phos have been described as being elevated in the mercury toxic patient due to the turnover of red blood cells. There are also some dietary factors which can elevate these two liver enzymes.

The foremost cause of an elevated LDH is sugar because the end result of sugar metabolism is lactic acid. This enzyme breaks down lactic acid. It can also be elevated by hard cheese and alcohol. The primary way in which we control LDH is to eliminate sugar and supplement with magnesium. If we are already giving liver enzymes for other liver function tests, they will work here as well.

Alk Phos is elevated dietarily by the use of alcohol.

So again, your responsibility in helping to correct your chemistries involves avoiding sugar and alcohol.

Let's look now at minerals (as seen in the hair analysis) whose activity is affected by mercury in the system. When we look at initial mineral levels on the first analysis, we can't be certain whether they are biologically active or not. If the level is in excess of the ideal level, we know that at least some of it is inactive. Our nutritional correction assumes inactivity when the level is too high and insufficient activity when the level is too low. Normally, the second test (made in about three or four months) will help us determine activity more accurately. We will discuss here only those minerals directly affected by mercury and what you can do to help your treatment progress more rapidly.

Triad: Calcium

Remember the triad described in our discussion of hair analysis? The most difficult combination to correct includes a high calcium. There are several ways this can be worsened nutritionally. The number one dietary cause of an elevated calcium is hard cheese. The second largest cause is milk and milk products (except butter). And third is the myriad of calcium supplements found on the shelves of drug stores and health food stores. Bonemeal and dolomite are two of the worst offenders. But nearly any supplement made of oyster shells or ground-up rocks will do the same thing. Many people are concerned about osteoporosis and take these calcium supplements in an effort to prevent it. However, we have observed in our patients that bone metabolism (specifically bone density) is controlled by the minerals, magnesium and manganese. These inactive forms of calcium serve to interfere with the absorption of the active forms of calcium, magnesium and manganese. In looking at patient chemistries, we find that without the interference of this inactive calcium, over 90 percent of our patients are able to absorb sufficient quantities of active calcium from the foods they eat. Though not a dietary source, a hard water supply can also affect the calcium level. If this is the case for you, we recommend the use of bottled water.

Why is it so important to avoid an elevated calcium level? Inactive calcium blocks the absorption and the action of active forms of calcium, magnesium, zinc, copper, iron and manganese. These minerals are extremely important in the system. A contaminant level of calcium has been related to cancer because it adheres to the outside of the cell membrane and causes interference with so many other nutrients in their efforts to get into and out of the cell.

Calcium is involved with the transmission of nerve impulses. Inactive calcium blocks and inactivates this impulse transmission so that it can act in a manner as an anesthetic to dull nerve impulses. This is one reason why taking calcium even when you have a contamination can stop menstrual cramps and leg muscle cramps. It has actually inactivated the transmission of those nerve impulses. But it has not solved the problem which is the deficiency of magnesium and manganese.

Calcium is highly influential in cell membrane metabolism, that is, in getting things into and out of the cell. When the inactive form goes into a cell, it tries to replace the other minerals as the key to the enzyme systems. But because it is not a key and cannot drive those systems, it causes imbalances. It can block thousands of enzyme systems at any given time.

Because both calcium and magnesium activate the process which begins the production of energy and because calcium is necessary for the absorption of magnesium, it is easy to understand that the proper amount of biologically active calcium at the cellular level is necessary for us to have a good energy level. Whether we have a deficiency of calcium or whether we have an inactive contamination makes no difference as far as the interference with this energy production. The result is still the same.

In summary, remember that calcium contamination can block the action of active calcium, magnesium, zinc, copper, iron and manganese. Approximately 90 percent of all the reactions in the body concern these minerals and their combinations. So if we are getting a source of inactive calcium, we are potentially interfering with 90 percent of the reactions in our body.

What about the triad which has a deficient calcium? This can be caused by diuretics (water pills and medications such as those given for high blood pressure) and by lecithin. It can also be caused by the loss of electrolytes through sweating (heavy exercise, hot climates, etc.).

Triad: Manganese

Perhaps the greatest negative dietary factor in the deficient manganese is alcohol. It acts as a diuretic and causes manganese to be excreted in the urine. There are not many causes of an elevated manganese other than over-compensation for mercury toxicity, but dietarily black teas and carrot juice can play a role.

The interruption of manganese metabolism is the greatest disturbance found in patients with such diseases as periodontal disease, arthritis, multiple sclerosis (MS), Muscular Dystrophy, cancer, heart disease and suicidal tendencies. Because of the continuous appearance of manganese deficiency in all degenerative disease, we consider it to be the most important factor in the degenerative disease profile. Its action is blocked first by mercury; next in line comes calcium. When both factors are present, you have doubled your susceptibility to any type of degenerative disease. Further, continual dietary insults to the body affect the endocrine system and the imbalance is more than can be overcome by the body.

A few of the functions of manganese are listed for you as follows:

> helps to control glucose level
> aids in the calcification of teeth
> works with magnesium to prevent muscle cramping
> aids in the development of the inner and outer ear

works with magnesium in the control of hyperkinetic and
autistic behaviour in children
aids nerve impulse transmission
helps prevent tingling and numbness in the limbs
works with zinc in the prevention of birth defects

After manganese is knocked out, your genetic code determines what disease you get. The symptoms of manganese deficiency come from the list above. Do they sound familiar to you? Have you already seen them in the list of symptoms of mercury toxicity?

Triad: Mercury

Though amalgams are the biggest source of exposure to mercury, they are not the only source. Dietarily we can *ingest* large amounts of mercury also.

Perhaps the greatest dietary source of mercury is canned tuna. This is followed closely by the shell fish like lobster and shrimp. As a rule, the larger the salt water fish, the greater the amount of mercury it contains. What is worse is that this is all *methyl* mercury. Mercury is methylated by bacteria and floats up into the plankton. Small fish eat the plankton and are in turn eaten by larger fish. Because the fish do not excrete very much of the methyl mercury (only 1 percent per day), the higher up the food chain you go, the larger the amount of methyl mercury.

Dr. Ben Lane in New York has shown a relationship between higher incidence of cataracts and the ingestion of fish more than once in two and one-half weeks. He relates this to the presence of methyl mercury.

Cell Membrane Permeability

There are several factors which influence the permeability of the cell membrane. Here we'll discuss only the trace minerals that are involved. The first two are calcium and manganese, which have already been discussed at length. The others are zinc, magnesium, chromium, sodium and potassium. Sodium and potassium are also involved in the transmission of nerve impulses and are quite often greatly out of balance in diseases like multiple sclerosis. Let's discuss the remaining minerals individually.

Zinc

Low levels of zinc can be caused by caffeine and alcohol while contaminations are caused by cheese and supplementation with inactive ingredients. One other important factor to be noted at this point is that zinc can be blocked by cadmium. Cadmium is found in margarine and is another reason why the mercury toxic patient should avoid it.

Zinc is essential in the activation of over 80 percent of the enzyme systems. Perhaps one of its most important functions is in helping to control glucose. As mentioned before, zinc is a part of the insulin molecule which is the control for glucose. It is also important in the growth of bone and along with magnesium is vital in the healing process. It is necessary in the development of all five senses so it is very important in the development of children. Keep this in mind during pregnancy when your dentists want to place an amalgam. Another extremely important function of zinc is the maintenance of healthy skin. Up to 20 percent of zinc is stored in the skin. When we see a patient with acne, we first think of zinc and those things which block its action — such as inactive calcium and mercury.

Zinc is necessary in sexual function and drive. This is one reason why when there is a lack of zinc for the development of a healthy fetus, there is usually no sex drive. Zinc along with manganese is extremely important in the prevention of birth defects. Zinc also helps to activate the hormones. Perhaps the interference with zinc and manganese activity is part of the reason why methyl mercury toxicity is so damaging genetically (100 times worse than Colchicine, acknowledged as the most damaging drug).

Zinc is also necessary in protein metabolism as well as in the control of pain postsurgically. But the primary function of zinc is the selective alteration of the permeability of the cell membrane. This means that it helps to selectively get nutrients into the cell.

Dietarily then, you should avoid hard cheese if your zinc level is elevated. And you should avoid sugar, alcohol and caffeine if your zinc level is deficient as seen in many mercury toxic patients.

Magnesium

A deficiency of magnesium can be caused by alcohol, by the birth control pill and by excess sugar consumption. On the other hand we can see inactive contamination levels of magnesium if there is a calcium contamination or if Dolomite is being used as a supplement. Magnesium is involved in the activation of 78 percent of all of the enzyme systems. Where we see a lack of magnesium, we see a higher decay potential so as a means of controlling dental decay, magnesium is essential.

Alcohol lowers magnesium levels because it is a diuretic. It alters kidney function in such a manner that neither magnesium nor zinc are reclaimed from the urine and sent back to the blood as they should be. Instead they are excreted.

What must you do to avoid problems with magnesium metabolism? If you have a low magnesium, you must avoid sugar, alcohol and caffeine. If you have an elevated magnesium, you must avoid milk, cheese and supplements like Dolomite and bonemeal.

Chromium

Low levels of chromium are found in the patient who eats large amounts of carbohydrate habitually, when there is a high manganese level and when there is a contamination with vanadium.

The reason why high intake of carbohydrate will lower the chromium is that chromium is necessary in the activation of insulin and is part of what is known as the Glucose Tolerance Factor. This works at the cell membrane to allow glucose to get into the cell. High levels of carbohydrates, especially sugar, increase the glucose level so that greater amounts of chromium are needed to metabolize it. When we have a low chromium level we have a difficult time controlling the glucose level. Therefore it is necessary to be very strict about dietary control and taking supplementation.

Potassium

Low levels of potassium can be caused primarily by medications such as cortisone, high blood pressure medications (these are diuretics), and the birth control pill. Nearly *all* medications and drugs will upset potassium metabolism. Alcohol and exercise can also cause potassium deficiencies. High levels are found when a patient is on Lite salt, kelp or sea salt. Lite salt is potassium choloride (KCl). It is especially bad about upsetting the fluid balance because it upsets the ratio between sodium and potassium. Kelp and sea salt have also been noted to upset this ratio.

Potassium deficiency and/or contamination is peculiar to MS patients as well as being the Number Two deficiency in the periodontal patient. We consider the balance between potassium and sodium to be extremely important. It is a balance that is extremely difficult to achieve. It takes a long time to build up a low potassium. If there is a contamination of inactive sodium and potassium, they usually drop drastically after the first analysis. These two minerals are especially noted for dropping even if the levels initially appear to be within Body Chemistry ideals because it is so easy to get contamination from inactive sources. The first hair tests are very seldom active minerals.

Sodium

We discussed some of the causes of excess sodium when we treated the subject of protein metabolism. But because this is so important to correcting chemistry imbalances, we will repeat it here.

Water softeners cause sodium to be metabolized differently, which is the reason why sodium from this source is biologically inactive. All soft drinks contain sodium benzoate. The "sugar free" soft drinks are sweetened with sodium saccharin. Preserved meats such as bacon and luncheon meats contain sodium nitrates, while fish are sprinkled with sodium nitrites. This process is cheaper than washing the fish with hot water to prevent botulism. MSG is monosodium glutamate and is a byproduct of the production of sugar. It is found in meat tenderizers and most seasoning salts as well as in Chinese food.

Bath beads contain such compounds as sodium laurelate which are absorbed through the skin and even more so in *hot* baths. Kelp not only causes sodium and potassium problems, but is a potential source of mercury as well. We have seen sea salt raise the potassium level and thus interfere with sodium metabolism. American-made soy sauces can cause problems with sodium levels, but the imported ones usually do not.

Margarine is the last source we will discuss. It contains sodium benzoate and cadmium which blocks zinc activity and is one of the leading causes of high blood pressure. It also fails to provide fat (like butter does) for the proper transport of nutrients. When looking at patients who use either margarine or no fats at all, we see problems. But the patient who uses margarine has more problems.

Summary of Foods to Avoid

Let's outline again those things which sould be avoided if you are suffering from mercury toxicity.

SUGAR

> raises serum glucose
> raises serum cholesterol
> raises serum triglycerides
> upsets endocrine balance
> depletes chromium
> depletes zinc
> depletes magnesium
> depletes manganese

ALCOHOL

> raises serum glucose
> raises serum cholesterol
> raises serum triglycerides
> raises alkaline phosphatase
> raises LDH
> upsets endocrine balance
> depletes magnesium
> depletes zinc
> depletes manganese
> depletes potassium
> interferes with protein metabolism if taken at meal time
> depletes folic acid which is also knocked out by mercury

CAFFEINE

> raises serum glucose
> raises serum cholesterol
> raises serum triglycerides
> raises uric acid
> upsets endocrine balance
> interferes with protein metabolism
> depletes magnesium
> depletes zinc

CHOCOLATE

> depletes chromium

MARGARINE

> contains cadmium — blocks action of zinc
> contains sodium preservatives — upsets sodium balance

SOFT DRINKS

> contain sugar, caffeine, sodium preservatives and sodium-containing artificial sweeteners

REFINED CARBOHYDRATES
        deplete chromium
        deplete manganese
        elevate glucose
        elevate cholesterol
        elevate triglycerides
        upset endocrine balance

MILK
        raises calcium level
        interferes with protein metabolism

CHEESE
        elevates LDH and other liver function tests
        elevates calcium
        elevates magnesium
        elevates zinc

LIQUIDS WITH MEALS
        interferes with protein metabolism

DOLOMITE, BONE MEAL, BONE MEAL SUPPLEMENTS
        raise calcium
        raise magnesium

INACTIVE SUPPLEMENTS
        raise any mineral level

LITE SALT   elevates potassium level

SALT WATER FISH
        contains methyl mercury

SMOKING
        not a food, but a negative nonetheless
        raises triglycerides
        raises cholesterol
        raises lead and nickel levels
        interferes with cell membrane metabolism —
           so slows excretion of mercury

And now which foods should you be sure *are* in your diet?

BUTTER
        To optimize cholesterol
        to enhance absorption of nutrients

EGGS
        to optimize cholesterol

SALT   to aid protein metabolism
                        to aid in transport of nutrients through the
                            cell membrane

PROTEIN   to stabilize glucose
                        to bolster immune system

CHAPTER VI

Mercury Sources Other Than Amalgams

As we've said many times now, amalgam is not the only source of mercury exposure. However, mercury toxicity can't be successfully treated until *all* amalgam is out of the mouth.

During the initial treatment phase it is important to avoid exposure to other sources of mercury. We are listing as many exposures as we know at the current time. Most of the them can be avoided quite easily. After initial treatment is completed and you are on a maintenance regimen, you may find that occasional exposure does not affect you severely. Just remember, though, that once you have been sensitized to something like mercury, you can always expect to have some type of reaction to any future exposure.

FOODS

Tuna — canned or fresh
Shellfish — shrimp, lobster, crab, oyster, etc.
Other large saltwater fish — swordfish, salmon, cod, etc.
Carrots
Lettuce
Grains treated with methylmercury fungicides — especially wheat
Kelp and other seaweeds

COSMETICS

Clairol hair dye
Mascara — water proof type especially
Skin lightening creams

MEDICATIONS & PERSONAL ITEMS

Preparation H
Toilet paper made from recycled paper
Calomel — body powders & talcs
Mercurochrome

Merthiolate
Laxatives containing Calomel
Psoriasis ointments
Calamine lotion
Contact lens solutions
Vaginal gels — especially those that are contraceptive

MISCELLANEOUS

Latex & solvent-thinned paints
Fabric softeners
Floor waxes & polishes
Air conditioner filters
Wood preservatives
Cinnabar — used in jewelry
Felts
Adhesives
Tatooing
Batteries with mercury cells
Sewage disposal
Fungicides for lawns, shrubs & trees

INDUSTRIAL

Bactericide makers
Barometer makers
Battery makers
Bronzers
Calibration instrument makers
Cap loaders, percussion
Carbon brush makers
Caustic soda makers
Chlorine makers
Dentists
Direct current meter workers
Disinfectant makers
Disinfectors
Drug makers
Electric apparatus makers
Electroplaters
Embalmers
Explosive makers
Farmers
Fingerprint detectors
Fireworks makers
Fish cannery workers
Fungicide makers

Fur preservers
Fur processors
Gold extractors
Histology technicians
Ink makers
Insecticide makers
Investment casing workers
Jewelers
Laboratory workers, chemical
Lampmakers, fluorescent
Manometer makers
Mercury workers
Miners, mercury
Miners, gold
Mirror makers
Neon light makers
Paint makers
Paper makers
Pesticide workers
Photographers
Pressure gauge makers
Refiners, mercury
Seed handlers
Silver extractors
Switch makers
Tannery workers
Taxidermists
Textile printers
Thermometer makers
Vinyl chloride manufacturers

You can see how many places mercury is used in our modern environment. It is impossible to avoid *all* sources, but you should make every reasonable effort you can. Read labels carefully and question every product mentioned in the list. There are usually acceptable substitutes for everything. For example, makers of contact lens solutions know that some people are "allergic" to the Thimerisol preservative (a mercury compound) used in their products. So there is at least one solution of every type (cleaning, soaking, etc.) for both hard and soft lenses that is preservative-free. Check with your ophthalmologist if you have need of these solutions.

This list should also be closely studied before you have the skin patch test for screening purposes so that you can avoid additional exposures during the course of the test and for a couple of days afterward.

CHAPTER VII

Dental Materials — The Good, The Bad And The Ugly

"Dental Materials" is a science in itself and now encompasses well over 1000 different metallic alloys to choose from. Metals are used in fillings, crowns, partial dentures, orthodontics and implants. Each company has its own formula for each item, with slight variations to avoid patent infringements.

Amalgam (The Bad and The Ugly)

The lay person tends to think of silver fillings as containing primarily silver, gold crowns as being nearly all gold and porcelain crowns as being made out of porcelain. For ease of communication, this terminology is employed. After all, who cares that a silver filling has tin, copper, zinc and mercury in it? It really wouldn't matter if these materials stayed put in the fillings. They don't. As they electrochemically slough off they become part of your body's biochemistry. Those that are poisonous create toxic reactions in your body. In a silver filling, toxic metals would include silver, copper, tin and — oh, yes — mercury.

As if "conventional" amalgam were not bad enough, there is now the very popular "high copper" amalgam. Chemically the high copper amalgams emit mercury 50 times faster than conventional amalgams. Clinically, when a person becomes ill due to high copper amalgam, it is extremely difficult (and many times impossible) to correct their disturbances. High copper amalgams should be entirely avoided even if you are personally not concerned about mercury toxicity. Ask your dentist what type of amalgam material he uses. Don't allow anyone to place high copper amalgam in your mouth or those of your family. Of all the metallic dental materials, high copper amalgam is probably the most deadly.

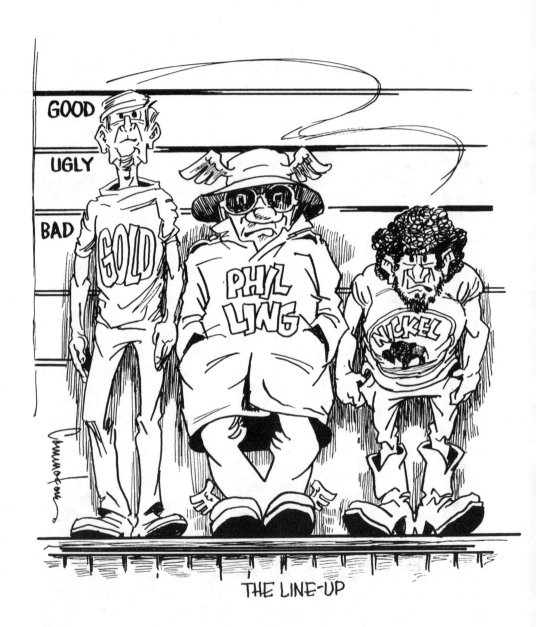

THE LINE-UP

Composites (The Good)

What can be used in place of amalgam? Is anything available that is comparable in cost and durability? The University of Colorado School of Dentistry studied the longevity of amalgam fillings and came up with this statement. The half life of amalgam is four years.

Interpretation: if 100 amalgams were placed today, 50 would still be in the mouth four years from now; 25 would still be in service eight years from now; 12 to 13 would still be there in 12 years and about six would still be left in 20 years.

Composites (filling materials made out of ground glass powder mixed with a plastic binder) require more time to place than amalgam, so the cost would be expected to run maybe 10 to 20 percent higher. Their life span is not known compared to the Colorado University study, but many have been noted to pass the five and ten-year mark. Manufacturers are improving composites each year. The whole concept boils down to one question. What's more important — the life of the filling or the life of the patient?

Composites come in two basic forms. Light-cure and chemical-cure. With the light cured materials, the material is placed into the tooth in a plastic form. A special light is concentrated on the material and causes it to harden in place. Chemically cured fillings consist of two pastes. When mixed together, a chemical reaction is set up which hardens the material.

Some people with allergies can tolerate the light-cure better than the chemical-cure due to the fact that the second continues to cure for a longer time than the first. Both materials seem to be suitable for 90 percent or more of the patients we see.

Gold (The Good)

All that glitters in your mouth may not be gold. Gold is relatively soft and in its pure state probably is not durable enough for long term wear. In the past years, other metals have been added not only to harden the gold but to reduce the cost. Platinum and palladium have been used to harden the metal, but now we find iridium, indium, gallium, silver and copper in "gold". Some "golds" contain less than 10 percent gold. The fewer the metals, the less complex the battery. So the higher the percentage of gold, the better the gold is for you biochemically. We've heard of a gold that is 90 percent gold and 10 percent platinum. That sounds great. Palladium appears to give a high current and so it becomes undesirable for that reason.

The metal we recommend is Stern's Bio-H (their "hard" crown and bridge gold) and Stern's Bio-C (metal for the base under porcelain crowns or "caps"). These may not be the best in the world, but they handle nicely and are currently considered the better ones as far as biocompatibility is concerned. We appreciate Stern Gold Company for having the guts to come out with a biocompatible material when the competition is specializing in cheap substitutes of nonprecious, toxic metals like nickel and beryllium.

Combinations of metal alloys create even more problems. Frequently badly broken teeth are "built up" with amalgam to furnish a post for the crown to sit on. As was shown earlier, gold over amalgam stimulates mercury deposition into the tissues adjacent to the root of that tooth.

When you are in the process of having your amalgams removed, be certain that final gold restorations are not placed until all amalgam is out. Temporary plastic crowns can be used to protect the teeth until all the mercury has been removed. Remember the problems that can occur when gold and amalgam are in the mouth simultaneously. (See abstract on Jaro Pleva's "Mercury Poisoning From Dental Amalgam" in appendix B.)

Nickel (Another Bad And Ugly)

Despite its known allergenic properties and toxicity, nickel has wormed its way into the biggest slice of the casting material market today. In some parts of the country, nickel is used in over 90 percent of the crowns made. Overall use is over 85 percent.

Nickel is used in place of gold to make crowns for badly broken down teeth when "cost is a factor". Its major use is as a base onto which porcelain is fired. This is how porcelain crowns or caps are made. Even though nickel is used in many removable bridges, the metal appears to be more detrimental in the form as used for crowns. Most of the adverse reactions are similar in toxicity to those of mercury. Neurological disturbances and blood problems (like leukemia) can be initiated by nickel crowns.

Many removable bridges (called partial dentures) are made of nickel. When we placed nickel partials in patients, we had to baby sit them for the first two weeks of "adjustments". Most people salivated more and

106

were conscious of having a horseshoe in their mouth. With persistence and understanding that it was just a matter of "getting used to it", we got along pretty successfully.

Strange, but the last two years of active wet-finger dentistry, we placed only gold partials. The cost was about $150 more (pass through on the actual gold cost) but they were thicker and heavier. Gold can be cast with amazing accuracy, so the fits were terrific. Patient reaction? Feels fine! No excessive salivation. No periodic removal while becoming adjusted. We wonder . . . does the body know that one is toxic and the other is not?

One thing we are beginning to note about nickel and other non-gold metals is that they create negative electrical current. Nickel and a palladium-silver-tin metal we have seen a lot lately have both registered negative current in some pretty sick patients.

So it saves you $20 or $30. Is it worth it? Ask the epileptic, the patient with multiple sclerosis or the leukemic counting his last days on earth. What a price to pay for economy!

If the patient selects it by choice, fine. O.K. We have no objection. We just don't want a dentist or anyone else making that kind of decision about our health without consulting us or giving us a choice. And we don't think any other patient should be denied the choice either.

Nickel has been used in children for several decades in the form of metallic preformed crowns used on badly decayed baby teeth. They are called "chrome or stainless steel crowns". Many of these emit negative electrical current. They set up a battery effect with amalgam in the mouth to make the mercury come out faster.

"Tin-grin" patients are showing off nickel, not tin. The amount of electrical current generated by "braces" is generally several times higher than that created by amalgam fillings. The current can be either positive or negative. We have even seen positive in one arch and negative in the other.

Allergists have told us that when they have a slightly allergic patient who is going to get braces, they brace themselves. They know that the allergies are going to get worse. Most of these doctors are not aware of the mechanism or they would have complained years ago. With the increase in electrical activity, all chemical reactions should proceed faster. This includes mercury coming out of the fillings, disrupting white blood cell metabolism and stimulating allergic reactions. Some of the worst reactions we have seen occurred where the patients had combinations of nickel, gold and amalgam — for instance when there were amalgam and gold restorations under orthodontic bands.

107

Bases

Metals conduct heat and cold faster than tooth enamel. This is one reason why teeth are sensitive to hot and cold changes after a new filling is placed. (Another reason is negative electrical current. Electricity can make teeth super sensitive for years.) In order to reduce the thermal shock from coffee and ice cream, etc., the dentist will frequently place a coat of insulation (called a "base") over the pulp chamber where the nerve lives. This has always been considered a very helpful thing to do for the patient's benefit. Now we are finding that Dycal, the most often used base material, gives many people the same reaction as mercury does. We have no idea why this is true, but enough patients have had to have their dentistry redone to make us hesitant to use or recommend it.

What is the best base? We don't know. Although it is not perfect either, we have found the best results overall with a base called Dropsin. It is available through most dental supply companies and is our choice until something better comes along.

Root Canals

Root canal fillings (that fill up the space formerly occupied by the nerve) can be done in two ways. Usually a hole is cut from the top of the tooth into the nerve chamber and the chamber is filled through the hole. Another method is used when the abscess is farther advanced. This involves cutting through the bone at the root end, cleaning out all the infected material there and then sealing the root tip and sewing the area together. Bone will fill in the defect. What material is usually used to seal the pulp chamber at the root tip? Amalgam.

"Retrograde filling" is the term applied to this type of root canal sealing process. Mercury now has direct access to the body fluids and can cause problems similar to those created from amalgam in the mouth. The only difference is that those fillings in the mouth are much easier to replace.

Special attention is paid to the patient with a retrograde filling. Certainly no one wants to go through that type of surgery twice unless there is a very good reason to do so. Usually all the other dentistry is done first and the patient is reevaluated.

SERVICES AVAILABLE THROUGH THE OFFICE OF
DR. HAL A. HUGGINS

You may write or call for information as listed below Monday through Friday. Our usual office hours are 8:00 a.m. to 12:00 p.m. and 1:00 p.m. to 5:00 p.m. We have an answering machine to record messages outside these hours.

Send self-addressed, stamped envelope with your request

1. Urinary excretion of mercury screening program

2. Computer diagnosis and treatment planning program for both mercury toxicity and nutritional evaluation

3. Information on becoming a patient in our practice of diagnosis and treatment planning. Dental work will be done by your personal dentist or by one from our referral list.

OFFICE TELEPHONE: (719) 473-4703
1-800-331-2303

If you wish to order information regarding the services we have available through our office, you may use this order form or call us. Our office hours are 8:00 a.m. — 12:00 p.m. and 1:00 p.m. — 5:00 p.m. Monday through Friday. An answering machine will take any messages for you if it is more convenient for you to call outside these times.

_____ Send me information about the screening program for urinary excretion of mercury.

_____ Send me further information about the computer program for diagnosis and treatment planning for mercury toxicity.

_____ Send me further information about becoming a patient in your practice.

Name _____

Address _____

City, State, Zip _____

Dr. Hal Huggins
P.O. Box 2589
Colorado Springs, CO 80901

Cleaning Teeth

The practice of cleaning teeth and polishing amalgam fillings can have an adverse affect. Cleaning the teeth presents no problem at all where there is no amalgam present. But the polishing procedure with pumice (done after the plaque and calculus or tartar are removed) removes a layer of corrosion from the amalgams. This increases the amount of mercury vapor coming off the fillings.

We have found that electrical current increases after polishing amalgams with a round bur. In fact, when we get no electrical reading with the Amalgameter on a corroded filling, we polish it to enable us to determine the polarity.

We're not saying that you shouldn't have your teeth cleaned — just that you should have your amalgams removed first. More and more of our patients are telling us that they have increased symptoms after having their teeth cleaned. It is certainly easy to understand why.

To recap dental materials, gold is best, costs most and lasts longest. Be careful to get a high quality gold, though. They are not all the same.

Composites are very low in electrical current, have no mercury, but don't wear as long as mercury-containing fillings. They cannot be used to restore cusps (the tips of the teeth on the chewing surface) any more than amalgam can. Large fillings should be crowned with gold.

Nickel is nearly as bad as mercury for those people who react to it. It is present in orthodontic bands, children's and adult's crowns, removable bridges and the base of procelain crowns.

There is a new generation of "cast glass" crowns, and some day inlays, coming on the market. From the standpoint of biocompatibility, they rank number one. There are mechanical limitations to these at the present time, but manufacturers are confident that they can perfect them if the need arises. Hopefully that need will arise by public demand shortly. If we were to need fillings placed today, we would prefer the cast glass type of restoration. You can help hasten the development by requesting these materials from your dentist today.

CHAPTER VIII

Treatment Summary — Getting Started
On The Road To Health

Now that you've read this far, we hope you have a clear understanding of the severity of mercury toxicity and the need for a properly planned treatment regimen. In this chapter, we are going to give you an outline of everything we've said so far. Please use it as you proceed with your plans for treatment.

STEP ONE

DO NOT HAVE YOUR AMALGAMS REMOVED WITHOUT GOING THROUGH ALL THE STEPS!!!!!

STEP TWO

If you're uncertain that mercury is a problem, have screening tests done.

Urine mercury — can be done for anyone. If not available in your area, can be done through our office.

Electrical reading of fillings — can be done for anyone. If not available in your area, see "Services Available" at the end of the book.

Skin patch test — be sure to understand exceptions to this test.

STEP THREE

Have electrical reading taken if not done in step two.

Have basic testing completed — CBC, profile, hair analysis, urine mercury if you have any symptoms or problems at all.

If you have no health problems, but are removing amalgams only for preventive reasons, you may be able to skip the testing, but be sure that you have the electrical readings done for sequential removal.

STEP FOUR

Start supplementation as determined by test results from step three at least one or two weeks before amalgam removal.

STEP FIVE

Have amalgams removed according to sequence as determined by electrical current. Do not use high palladium gold as a replacement filling.

Do not have gold placed before all amalgam is out.

Do not have crowns permanently cemented for at least one month if your symptoms are severe.

Do not use bases like Dycal.

Follow nutritional guidelines.

Avoid other mercury exposures.

Avoid having all appointments on the same day of the week in order to avoid interfering with the 21-day immune cycle.

***If suicidal thoughts are part of your symptoms:

Be sure PZI (protamine zinc insulin) is used with each quadrant of amalgam removed.

Have someone stay with you for the first 24 hours after treatment; the more negative current you have, the more important this is.

If you are unable to find someone who can plan your treatment and are unable to come to our office, we can still help you with a computer program designed specifically for this purpose. You may contact our office for further information. There should be no reason for anyone suffering from mercury toxicity to be unable to find help.

Finally we want to ask your help in getting this problem eliminated. Write the ADA, write the FDA. Write Congressmen Tim Wirth and Henry Waxman (see Chapter IX for their addresses). Make your opinion known that mercury is unsafe to be used in dentistry. With your help the problem *can* be solved.

Follow-Up Testing and Lifestyle Requirements

After the diagnosis is made and the treatment plan designed, then what? Supplementation, sequential removal, dietary changes. Now what is going to happen? It's like shooting at a target over the hill. How do you know if you hit the target?

That's what the follow-up chemistry is all about. Symptom changes are the bottom line for you personally. You want to have more energy, stop having seizures, feel good about life instead of being depressed. But you need scientific guidelines too, or *you* can decide its "all in your head".

Blood profile, CBC, hair analysis and urinary excretion are the basic tests used to determine the extent of problems. If progress is being made, these chemistries should change for the better.

Diagnosis is based on these chemistries, but from the research we have done in 18 other areas, we know these are not *all* the changes that take place. The four "basics" give us an affordable analysis that covers the major areas of imbalance, though not every imbalance. If an outlying factor is at fault, then the basic chemistries are not likely to respond. Fortunately, chemistries that don't respond usually point toward the area of interference, and we can figure out where to look next.

For the most part, follow-up involving three of the four initial tests gives us a good overview of progress. The CBC, blood profile and urine mercury excretion can show significant changes in anywhere from just a few days to three weeks. So we get a good, quick, inexpensive indication of progress. At the present time we look at follow-up tests on our patients three weeks after amalgam removal has been completed.

The first area of concern is urinary excretion of mercury. If low excretions have not come up, we do not expect much change in the other chemistries. This is the time to reassess the original chemistries and the diet to see if something was overlooked or if the patient is really following the dietary recommendations and avoiding other exposures. The most common problem seems to be that the patient is still consuming caffeine.

Since supplementation is originally designed as conservatively as possible, the patient may not be taking enough of a particular supplement to activate the mercury excretion mechanism. The supplementation regimen will then be altered to meet the patient's needs.

Next we look to the CBC. Since fatigue is a major factor in so many people, hemoglobin and hematocrit levels are of primary concern. They may improve by either going up or down. That sounds illogical until we rethink the chemistry. If hemoglobin is saturated with mercury and the body's compensatory mechanism is producing high amounts of hemoglobin, we have fatigue. If enough mercury is removed to allow a normalization of hemoglobin level with uncontaminated hemoglobin, then a lowering of the excessive level usually points to energy increase.

White blood cells are a prime factor in people whose immune system is not up to par. At three weeks, several swings have taken place and a pseudostability may have occurred. Dozens of changes can happen here as each of the individual types of white cells can go up, go down or some even disappear. Each of the various combinations of up and down carries a different interpretation. The excitement associated with these changes is more intense in the CBC than in any of the other chemistries because immune response determines overall health.

Blood serum chemistry is partly mercury-related and partly related to nutrition. This is the most complex area to interpret in follow-up for that reason. All the other chemistries plus diet and lifestyle play a role in altering the values of glucose, cholesterol, triglycerides, total protein, etc. This doesn't mean that it is impossible to interpret, just that each factor has to be weighed against the other factors known to produce changes. For the most part, when the body has an opportunity to heal (as with the removal of a toxin like mercury) all systems work together to produce a better, healthier body. This produces predictable changes in the chemistry and an outlying factor is easy to spot. Outliers sometimes require special attention.

How long do you have to remain on a good diet and take supplements? Once the body has been challenged with mercury and lost the battle (you got sick!) it is more susceptible to recurrence than is your neighbor's who didn't get sick. The answer could be, as long as you want to be in better health. A good diet is a good idea for anyone. Supplementation is often necessary for basic correction, but not always necessary forever. If you have access to "organically" grown foods and good water, you may be able to derive all of your nutritional needs from your foods. If your body has sustained some direct blows and needs more of a particular substance than is available in a normal diet, supplementation may be required for an indefinite period.

This is where follow up with the hair analysis comes in. After you have had your amalgams removed, have made alterations in your diet, have avoided excess mercury exposure and have been on supplementation for three or four months, a repeat hair analysis will let you know what is happening within the cells over an extended period of time. In other words, it will let you know what your new lifestyle is doing for you. It will enable you to further refine your diet and your supplementation based upon your current needs. We personally check our own chemistries about once every six months and recommend this for all our patients.

Even without a hair analysis, though, maintenance supplementation can be good preventive medicine. It will not cause imbalances. Maintenance in our practice usually consists of TransMix to enhance generalized absorption, vitamin C for a number of reasons and X-IT for the "rainy day". Optional supplementation includes digestive enzymes where the body continues to need help and Vitamate for a well-balanced, daily vitamin-mineral combination that does not overdose any area.

Beyond this, we prefer to be able to monitor and prescribe for your needs on the basis of chemistry excesses and deficiencies (which we see primarily in the hair analysis). There are a few exceptions, of course. Vitamin E is fine up to 400 units daily. Some people react adversely above that figure. Multiple vitamins are okay as long as the vitamin B-12 does not exceed 10 micrograms daily. More than this amount depletes the body of folic acid which is one of the primary vitamin deficiencies created by mercury toxicity.

We hope that we have given you a complete picture of the destructive potential of mercury toxicity and have enabled you to feel the anger and frustration we feel each time we see a patient who has been devastated by the mercury in "silver" fillings. But more than this, we hope we have given you a clear picture of how you can help yourself if this book has described your problems.

If we could say only one thing to you, it would be, "Don't have any more mercury or nickel placed in your mouth."

If we could make one request of you it would be that you tell everyone you know about what you have read here, including Congressmen Wirth and Waxman so that mercury, as used in dental fillings, can be taken off the market as soon as possible. And remember above all else that if you are going to have your fillings removed and replaced with a safer material that you *do it right the first time*. Remember to start supplementation prior to amalgam removal; to have your fillings removed in the proper sequence according to their electrical current readings; and to observe the dietary rules neccessary to help you excrete the mercury stored in your body's cells. And finally, if you can't find help in your area in which you feel confident, contact our office. We will help you find a dentist who will work with us and will guide you both step-by-step through the intracacies of treatment. Maybe your problems are *All In Your Head*, but perhaps they are limited to the lower half which contains those common silver-mercury amalgam fillings which you now know all about. We wish you success in your search for good health. God bless you all.

Honorable Henry A. Waxman
Chairman Subcommittee on
Health & Environment
2415 Rayburn House Office Bldg.
Washington, DC 20515

Congressman Timothy Wirth
2454 Rayburn House Office Bldg.
Washington, DC 20515

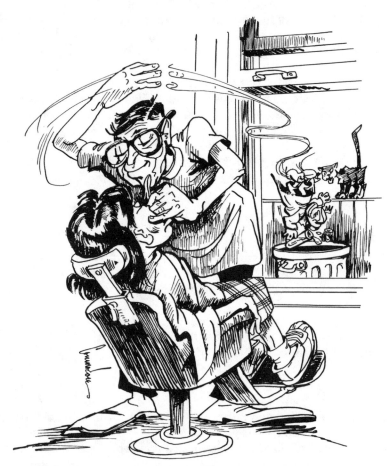

THAT'S THE CAVITY MERCURY AMALGAM SHOULD FILL

APPENDICES

Description Of The Problem
Through Case Histories

This chapter is a departure from the usual presentation of case histories. We have been asked again and again to present our patients as statistics and numbers. How many MS patients have you treated and how many got well? Show proof that all the chemistries you have been doing show exactly the same thing on each patient. Where are your double blind studies?

Well, we feel that it is time that our patients be known for what they are — people. People whose lives have been affected by mercury amalgams. If we could show you the videotapes we have of most of our patients, your tears would join ours as you see their pain and suffering.

This chapter is taking the place of our videotapes. Both Hal and I have our "favorite" patients — those whose lives we keep up with a little more than others. We didn't know how to write these stories any other way except just to tell them to you as if you were here with us. Throughout the rest of the book, we have both had our say in all the chapters. We have combined our joint experiences to bring everything together for you. But in this chapter, we are "going it on our own" with our special cases.

KD

We base our treatment on numbers. Each chemistry report comes to us as a number. We even talk in numbers. We might say, "Remember Don's 235? It's now 176. And that lymph of 1? It's now 21. Wow!"

No way can one feel the emotion that we felt — or that he felt. The one thing numbers can't tell the world is how mercury has affected people's lives. Some numbers are important. They are the way the academic community communicates. We use them, too.

What was his 235? It was 235,000 white blood cells. It was leukemia. Normal is 5,000-10,000. Within less than 48 hours after amalgam removal his white count was down to 176,000. A drop of nearly 60,000 cells from Thursday afternoon til Saturday morning. That's okay, but the lymphs were the big story. Lymphocytes are good fighters against chronic myologenous leukemia (CML). He was a CML'er. On Thursday he had 1 percent lymphs. The highest he had had since onset of CML was 9 percent and that was due to an intravenous injection of a powerful drug for that purpose. His lymphs in the absence of amalgam had skyrocketed to 21 percent. The dignified, terminal MD before me melted into tears. He cried for half an hour. I cried with him.

Was his terminal leukemia due to his fillings? It started within weeks of having a nickel crown and nearly a dozen amalgams placed. Time seemed like molasses. Was it a fluke? Would it continue? Could this be the answer for him and thousands more leukemia patients? We don't know. That was yesterday as I write this. He, Sharon, my staff and I will hold our breath until next Monday for the next blood test. Hope. Prayer. Thanksgiving. Doubt. All these emotions run through us.

How many times in the past have we held our breath over suicide, multiple sclerosis, epilepsy, migrains . . . how many times? Do we always win? No, but as we learn more, the percentage of success creeps up. So many peoples' lives are affected. So many people you will never see. They suffer in silence at home. No one wants to hear about desperation, terminal diseases, hopelessness and death. We don't mind them when they have a happy ending. But why must we have so many horror stories when they could be eliminated by changing the minds of half a dozen men — scientists who say that none of this happens. It doesn't happen in *their* lives. I want to beseech God to remove KD's leukemia and plant it in the families of those stubborn men quaking for their jobs. When leukemia hits their families, they may listen. If not, may they spend one year in hell for each person who has become ill due to amalgam since 1974. Or how about starting the time at the year they became aware that mercury comes out of fillings? That was 1969. Am I too cruel? How about if I ask all of the patients in this book? How about it, you millions of people who suffer a little or alot because of a few mens' negligence? Too emotional? Come walk in my moccasins for a day. Meet these people. Some of them are your neighbors. Some are you.

Hal just said what we both feel on a daily basis. Several months ago, I would not have agreed to let statements such as he has made above appear in writing. But this time I agree with him. I went with him to Chicago to try to convince those men that amalgam should be pulled off the market until more testing can be done to prove that what we are saying is true. They would not listen. They had their minds made up before Hal ever delivered our presentation. Yes, they do deserve to feel the pain and the devastation that amalgam causes so that they will take a fresh look at the possibility of getting rid of this health hazard. They need to feel what our patients feel so that they will not think of them only as numbers.

WA

WA's father sat beside her while her muscles went into violent spasms. She was awake. She was staring off into space wishing she weren't there. Her father felt each spasm. He was not quite stoic, but calm. He had witnessed thousands of these seizures in the past three months. Now this eleven-year-old girl's body was being lashed by its own muscles for five minutes every fifteen minutes. She couldn't walk, couldn't stand, could hardly talk or think. Six months ago she was an active, straight-A student. Now she took an average of 90 seconds to answer even the simplest addition problem. Eight thousand dollars worth of medical testing had sentenced her to a mental institution. Incidently, both parents were told they needed psychotherapy. It was "all in her head".

Yes, I agreed, all in her head. All these seizures had started a month after two small negative current fillings were placed. We didn't know whether fillings were the problem or not. Negative electrical current was a new discovery at that time. Is there any way to scientifically measure what she had gone through this past three months? How does it feel to have your body take over and leave you powerless to direct its functions? What are thoughts of death like to an eleven-year-old?

What is it like to see your daughter disintegrate before your eyes? Do you still love your sister when she gets all the attention and is an embarrassment to everyone? How do you test that? What's the normal range? I saw it all — right there in her father's eyes.

Yes, we'll remove the fillings.

We had a calculated fifteen minutes in which to remove three negative current fillings (one had been in prior to the two that broke the camel's back neurologically). Sharon and I worked with hardly a word. We had no time to speak. We had to think to each other. It can be done when you have to. Three amalgams out and three composites in. Then it hit. I've already described in the first chapter the way she took four of us (over 600 lbs total) and threw us around like rag dolls with the seizure which followed the amalgam removal.

How could the ADA have said that we "faked" what this child went through?

I told her I wanted her for my Christmas present. That was December 19th.

"What do you think?" Sharon asked as they drove off.

"I don't know."

We never know. We see people who don't deserve their misfortunes come in with suggestive chemistries. We design the treatment the best we know how, but bottom line is, we don't know. We wait.

On December 25th, whe woke up. Her numbness and paralysis from the neck down was gone. She got out of bed, walked downstairs by herself and never had another seizure.

What was Christmas like statistically?

In May of the next year we videotaped WA doing the 100 yard dash in 14.8 seconds. She was never institutionalized. Her parents never had psychotherapy.

ADA official reaction: "We're not impressed."

Now that Hal has repeated his story of WA for you, I have my turn. She was my first experience with severe neurological problems. Her dad was my first experience with "I won't take no for an answer!" The family was a very strongly religious family. Perhaps this is one of the reasons why they felt there was something more to her problems than just sibling rivalry.

When her dad brought her in to the office, he needed help getting her up the stairs. I was available. I'm no weakling but I could hardly hold her as we brought her up. I could hardly believe that she was only 11 years old. Such strength!

We wanted to capture her seizures on videotape so that after her recovery we could show others the difference. We find that this is the best way to help someone understand the severity of the problem. I still get chills throughout my whole body everytime I see the tape — or even think about — the seizures I watched that morning. Such a sweet child lying there on the couch and being jerked so uncontrollably. Can you imagine what it was like to someone so young to see herself on the television monitor as the tape rolled? But she was a real trooper. And she wanted to be able to help others in the future.

I cannot possibly describe the elation I feel when I think of her running at track meets now. And I get livid thinking of what she would be like right now if she had been institutionalized! Dentistry, please wake up! See what mercury can do to so many children — and adults — like WA. Please discontinue using amalgam!

BD

BD was suicidal. No particular reason, just once in a while suicide seemed like a good idea. Sort of like tying a shoelace that had come untied. Her family knew about this quirk. Four psychiatrists knew about it. She couldn't be watched 24 hours per day, so everyone knew that some day she would succeed — and not even know she was doing it.

I had known her for 15 years. I had watched her and her family as her children grew from grade school into college. I never suspected. One day she asked for help. She asked if Body Chemistry could do anything for her. It sounded mercurial to me, so I checked the fillings. You guessed it. Negative electrical current. Now, guess again. Who do you suppose put those fillings in her mouth 15 years ago?

We carefully removed the two worst offenders. She left the office to go home. Then she altered her path home. Suddenly a good idea came to her. It was time to commit suicide.

Alone and at the last second she remembered that she had left an important letter unanswered. She decided that the letter took precedence. How close!

Now we see that every suicidal patient (the second largest section of our practice) has someone with them every second for 24 hours after the initial amalgam removal. PZI (Chapter 15) administered immediately after the initial removal of negative fillings has pretty well prevented such occurrences. But we don't take chances any more.

BD was involved in several emotionally trying experiences over the next year, but took them in stride.

"I can cope now," was her comment. She didn't like the traumas that befell the family, but, "we can sure work them out" was her attitude. It has held for over two years.

Why is suicide the second biggest part of our practice? That bothers me. Our thought goes back to methyl mercury. Within minutes of leaving the filling, mercury can methylate and be incorporated into the brain.

Suicidal thoughts hit different people in different ways. It usually creeps in without warning. There is a common denominator. Patients usually don't tell their family or friends. I try to get them alone and tell them I see a chemical pattern that I've seen in people with weird suicidal thoughts. Thoughts not related to hating mother, daddy, the kids or the job. They usually pale and gasp. Relief infiltrates into their bodies as they realize that this may be toxicity and not a mental deficiency.

Religion plays a distinct role here. Some religions criticize suicide more than others. For those people whose religions are very strict about suicidal thoughts, the poor patient experiences a living hell because there is no one they feel they can discuss their problem with. They bear their guilt alone.

HL

We have been 100 percent successful at "curing" some diseases and have had 100 percent failures with other diseases. The diseases which fall into these categories are the ones where we have only one patient case history for each disease. This is one of the "100 percenters".

HL had been everywhere. No one could figure out what he had, except "HL's Disease". Many diseases surprise us, but this was and still is one of the most unusual. At first I didn't believe him, but then be began to show us the artifacts. He either petrified or dissolved his clothes depending on whether they were cloth or leather. His perspiration would dissolve the temple pieces of his glasses. He had gold-plated temple pieces made. Only the strongest acids will dissolve gold. He took off his glasses and showed them to us. They *were* dissolving. Gold was rusting! I know something about chemistry and had a hard time believing what we were seeing. Yet here were the glasses sitting on the desk.

He took his leather billfold out of his pocket. The part closest to him was solidified. It had petrified. His belt was the same. A belt only lasted two weeks for him. His perspiration would dissolve the underarms of a shirt in two days. But these things didn't hurt.

That's not why he was here. His body in the area of his undershorts was a mass of fiery blisters. He couldn't stand, sit or lie down without excruciating pain. A bowel movement was unbearable. Salves, ointments, creams, steroids, antibiotics — nothing had given any relief. He was suicidal, but not the ethereal "wander-in-and-out-of-the-mind" type. It was the "this-is-more-than-I-can-stand" type. He was a strong — a really strong — man. He could lift 200 pounds easily. Stories of his unflinching demeanor on the farm when other men would scream in pain were legends. Not on this day. He was brought to his knees.

We wasted little time in getting analyses done. This was one of the few times we found an elevated mercury in the blood. Most of the levels we had been seeing were 6-8 micrograms per liter. He had 13 mcg — nearly double. As fast as the blood clears mercury, we figured he had had a sizable exposure. That was only part of the problem. His lead level (as seen in the hair analysis) was 36 ppm, where 0-12 ppm is acceptable. Cadmium was 4.4 ppm, where less than 0.8 ppm is desirable. Heavy metals were accumulating and his ability to excrete them was down.

Today we can see other features that were there then, but we just didn't know how to interpret them at that time. He was extremely fatigued. His red cell count was 6 million (quite high), hematocrit was 51.6 percent (very high) and hemoglobin was 17.6 (quite high). Today we immediately think of mercury contaminating the hemoglobin binding sites as described earlier.

At that time — September, 1980 — we weren't sure what to think about amalgam removal for a case like this one. We did Body Chemistry balancing procedures first and probably through increasing the body's ability to excrete heavy metals were able to help him appreciably.

Within a month, he was markedly improved, but still had problems. Four months later we decided to get the amalgams out to see if the fillings were hindering progress. They were. As soon as they were removed, all his symptoms disappeared.

There are many people who stay on their prescribed nutritional program 85 percent of the time. Not HL. Ask him how closely he follows it and he will tell you 100 percent in such a fashion that you have not the slightest doubt that he is telling the truth. Besides, he's big!

When visiting relatives out of state a year ago, a neighbor came over to the relative's house. Since HL was visiting from Colorado and the neighbor was a dentist who had just heard a dentist from Colorado speak at a dental meeting, a comment was made. It went something like, "I just heard a dentist from Colorado tell us that amalgam is not good. How could anyone be so wrong?"

As I understand it, HL "levitated" this gentleman a foot off the floor with one hand and calmly explained why he thought that dentist from Colorado was right. By the time the dentist touched ground again, he was not inclined to criticize the speaker from Colorado. It seems that personal experience makes the difference in people's perception of whether or not mercury is poisonous.

WC

WC had a typical collage of problems that culminated in her having to reduce her concert schedule. She is one of the top (if not *the* top) performers in her field. Musicians need hands and she was losing control of hers. This had created some embarrassing moments on stage and even though she was at the apex of her career, it looked as if she would have to stop. This was heartbreaking.

Tracing history sometimes shows a path. Let's look backwards in time starting with the current problem. What's the problem? Arthritis. Painful, swollen joints. Muscle tenderness. Not conducive to hours of rehearsals. What about last year? Anything different about last year?

Yes. Tachycardia had started. Remember that this is where the heart races quite fast. Her heart would wake her out of a sound sleep and feel like it was doing flip-flops.

Anything before that? Well, yes. The year before that her memory began to slip badly. Again, not good for a musician. More? Yes, a yeast infection called *Candida albicans*. Now listen in on our initial appointment.

"Did anything stimulate the *Candida*?"

"Yes, it started as a result of a reaction to an antibiotic."

"What was the antibiotic given for."

"Pains and swelling in my hands. It turned out to be arthritis, but at that time the doctor thought it might be an infection."

"What happened before that?"

"I began stuttering. I had never stuttered before and at that time I was well into my thirties."

"Anything before that?"

"Yes. A possible diagnosis of lupus erythematosis. It was never really confirmed, but the doctor thought that's what I had."

"Before that?"

"I had a bad case of mononucleosis."

"Was that related to anything? Stress, long hours or anything like that?"

"I had just had a root canal and a lot of dental work. That's when the fatigue hit me first. My hands began to be achy and stiff and I ran a high white blood cell count for a long time."

"Before that?"

"I had always been quite healthy."

This case could be any of hundreds we have seen. It is typical to see one problem lend itself to another while the patient makes a pilgrimage from doctor to doctor. If your short term memory is working well you may remember having most of these symptoms presented in other parts of the book as being related to mercury toxicity.

What did the chemistry say at the time she came to see us? What was her electrical current? The white cells were still elevated. They were 9300. Her red cells, hemoglobin and hematocrit were low. To us this indicates long-term fatigue. The initial reaction of mercury in the hemoglobin is a compensatory elevation of cells. Then after the cell-producing mechanism grows tired, production drops off. Her production was off.

Her body temperature ran 97.2-97.4 degrees F. Does that tell us something? You bet. Many (not all) mercury toxic patients run low temperatures.

Let's look in the mouth. Do we expect to find mercury? Of course, that's what this book is all about. Two fillings. But one thing that might be a factor peeped out from behind the nice looking procelain bridge. A silvery, shiny metal was showing through the porcelain on the tongue side. That is normal procedure. Porcelain is placed where you can see it and the metal is left exposed on the inside where you can't see it. It's like white sidewalls on tires. The white is only on the outside.

Let's check this situation with the Amalgameter. The two amalgams were +3 and +5. Not too good, not too bad — sort of non-committal.

Then by the porcelain to metal bridge I spotted some purple spots. These were amalgam tatoos. Mercury and other heavy metals had been electrolytically deposited in her gums next to the bridges. Next we checked the shiny bridge metal. Negative 10, negative 8. The other bridge — negative 28. A crown — negative 25. The problem was now apparent. With all that negativity — and quite high at that — mercury was being pulled out. Nonprecious metals of some kind were being pulled out. And if my theory is correct, negative current was producing more methyl mercury. Methyl mercury has an affinity for sulfur groups on red cells, white cells and nervous tissue. All of a sudden the whole scenario unfolded and one disease blended into another, until we didn't have a dozen different problems. Just one. Toxic metals.

Yes, the story has a happy ending. The silvery metal bridges (possibly nickel according to the dentist who placed them) and the amalgams were removed. Her energy came back (red cells went up, hemoglobin went up, hematocrit went up), her fingers began to work again, the swelling in her knuckles went down, she lost four pounds and her cholesterol dropped over 100 points. Oh, yes. She gave a great concert. All this in less than two months.

Where did it start? In the dental office.

Where did it stop? In the dental office.

CP

Allergies affect different people in different ways. People affect people in different ways, too. CP was that way. She was a universal reactor who couldn't be around chemicals that most people aren't even aware of. She had an added problem. She didn't have enough balance to walk. Neighbors began to talk about her being an alcoholic. That was a laugh! One drop of alcohol would probably do her in. How nice, though, to have neighbors think such nice thoughts.

After amalgam removal she wrote to us: "I can't tell you how refreshing it is from being laughed at and looked at and treated like a freak."

We tried to work with her and her husband via long distance and the computer program. Any dentist should be able to follow the computer program. Her dentist didn't bother to read the directions with the

Amalgameter we sent to him. "If fillings are severely corroded the meter will not pick up a current. Take a round bur and cut off the corrosion layer. Then you can read the current."

The dentist touched several fillings, got no reading, took another look at her and told her not to bother. "Go home and make your peace with God. This won't do you any good anyway."

Thanks for the death sentence.

She and her husband (one of the most caring husbands I have ever seen) went home. Home was not the sort of thing you see in "House Beautiful". All linoleum and wall covering had to be torn off to the bare wood. She was not allergic to wood. Bamboo mats were on the floor for her to crawl on. It was easier on her hands and knees than raw wood.

He can go to hell; I'm going to Colorado.

Now, going to Colorado is not just an 800 mile trip. There are highway fumes to be contended with, but just like Dr. MA, they did it at night. Where can you stay in Colorado Springs that is "environmentally safe"? Nowhere, except in the car in our parking lot. Oh, I forgot to mention, it was winter! She and her husband slept in their car for several nights while her dentistry was being done. I remember the first evening when Sharon and I drove off to our warm home. We both looked back at that young couple in the snow-covered car and cried. God, how can you allow dentists to keep doing this to people? I thought of the ADA's pompous comments, "There is no documented evidence." Sleep in the snow. The ADA doesn't care. They don't laugh at you, they just say you don't exist.

It was hard to go home, but there was no other way. They were happy. They had hope.

The next morning two dentists and a television crew watched as her husband and I carried her into the dental office of Dr. Greg Mock, the young, caring dentist who helps us with patients like this. The next day one of the dentists was aghast to see her walking upright into the office. He has been very supportive ever since. The other one still won't speak to us.

Tom Beardon from Denver's Channel 7 was on the scene the first day as we carried her in. Discretely hidden, but keenly observing. He has interviewed, videotaped and followed many patients, never violating a privacy. His genuine interest in the health of the public is far greater than any medical or dental society I have seen. When amalgam is finally laid to rest somewhere other than in peoples' mouths, Tom Beardon will have had a big hand in bringing it about. Probably through public awareness. Thank you in advance, Tom, and all your patient camera men — bearded and otherwise.

CP is getting stronger by the day. Those temporary fillings Dr. Mock placed have lived up to their name. They were supposed to last two months. It's been nine. They are coming back to Colorado Springs to have him place composites. This time she will walk into the office under her own power. She won't spend the night in a snowbank, either.

I have to add my two cents worth, too. We've said several times that dentists are caring, concerned individuals. For the most part this is true. But why do people like this young woman have to run across the exceptions? I will never forget the day we received a call from Sandy, our receptionist. Hal and I were at a professional seminar in Palm Springs, enjoying the relative peace and quiet — a welcome break from the hectic schedule we follow at home.

A message was given to me that I should call the office immediately. There was an emergency. When I got Sandy on the phone, she was in tears and angry! She related the story about CP's experience with the dentist. CP was about ready to give up and die. Sandy gave me the telephone number, and I called CP. I had only a few moments between lectures, but I felt the need to talk to her personally. Her reaction to my call was one of gratitude and renewed hope. We decided that upon my return to the office, I would make arrangments to have her dental treatment done by Dr. Mock. How little it really took to give back the desire to live.

RL

We first examined RL in January, 1983. She was one of our few house calls. She was a universal reactor and couldn't come into town to see us. She lived in a stainless steel trailer away from humanity. She could eat only limited foods and those only one at a time. Sound familiar?

She was 28 years old and faced a lifetime of seclusion. Somehow we felt that her lifetime would be short, though, if we couldn't help her — suicide was an ever present threat.

129

Getting records on RL was difficult. We couldn't be inside her trailer without wearing special clothes, so we examined her outside in the snow. Hal and I tried to get Amalgameter readings, but the meter began to freeze up after about 10 minutes. We were able to determine that she had negative current in one very large filling, though.

Hal tried to draw her blood for the Profile and CBC, but the blood froze in the needle and we couldn't get the amount we needed for the test. She couldn't take the questionnaire into the trailer with her because she would react to the ink on the paper, so I took her health history through the rear window. What a sight — the two of us yelling at each other through the window! But we did find it amusing and enjoyed each other immensely throughout the whole procedure.

We went to work trying to set up a treatment plan for her. This would involve scheduling a Sunday in the dental office (we were still doing dentistry at that time, so Hal and I were going to do the work), arranging for a paramedic team to be on standby in case she had a reaction to anything, lining up her immunologist to be available in case we needed him and lining up the dental technician to make the gold crown we needed. Then there were the other "little" things like finding 100 percent cotton clothes for both Hal and me!

We contacted some friends at two gold companies, because after testing we found that she was one of the rare patients who could not have composites. Williams Gold Company donated the gold foil we needed to replace the smaller fillings and Stern Gold Company donated the gold we needed for the crown. God bless you for your help. You see, RL had been through so many diagnostic and treatment programs for her illness that she and her parents were nearly bankrupt. We were doing her case for only a token charge of $250. But it was almost more than they could handle. They would never have been able to afford the gold — and in our financial condition we couldn't have done it either. But you know, there are times when no matter what it takes, things have to get done. It was this way with this young lady.

Her parents drove her into town "strapped" to an oxygen tank. She arrived in good spirits and nearly died laughing when she saw the two of us in our "safe" garb. We started in on her treatment — without anesthetic. Her physician was concerned that anything we could give to numb the teeth would kill her. I don't know how she got through the nine long hours required to do all of her treatment!

She taught us something — as all of our patients do. As each amalgam was removed, one tooth at a time, she went through a series of reactions. We had never experienced anything like this before and didn't even recognize what was happening until about the third time it occurred. As each filling was removed (down to the last little speck) she would feel faint, feel that she was going to choke to death, salivate heavily, become extremely cold to the touch and wet on herself. Those we could all handle. What just about undid everyone was the personality changes she would go through. Talk about split personalities! She would change intermittently from the loving, strongly religious person we knew to a veritable bear with foul language and mean, viscious thoughts about us. What a day for all of us!

Somehow we all survived that day. The next morning we called to see how she was doing. Her mom was encouraged, but had a lot of questions. Why was she urinating so profusely, day and night? Where did all that fluid come from? She hadn't been drinking anything. And so on . . .

Here it is, one and one-half years later and where is RL? The last time we spoke to her she was able to live in Denver and was contemplating marriage. What a change from the total isolation she had previously faced. Her recovery was a long, hard road. She had many setbacks and wanted to commit suicide several times. Her strong faith pulled her through that. I can't count the number of hours I spent talking with her, trying to give her encouragement and trying to help her remember how bad she had been to begin with.

This is typical of many of our patients. Once they begin to get better, they forget how bad they were at the start. The setbacks are worse because they have had a taste of getting better. But this is extremely important for every mercury toxic patient to remember. There will be bad days as well as good days until your body has a chance to recover biologically in all the necessary areas.

Where Sharon came up with her innovative ideas is still a mystery. Each time RL would call it was a different type of crisis, but at least she called us instead of "doing something". I could handle the technical aspects of what was happening and explain them satisfactorily to her. But the other things . . . When she was confused and irrational my words got garbled, too. Sharon could slip into the conversation and have RL thinking and figuring things out for herself within a few minutes. Sharon's influence would last for about two days, then a new onslaught would erupt. Fear, anger, loving, resolved to dying, enthusiastic about living, hating the world, hating herself, worrying about her past, worrying about her future. Instinctively Sharon would speak in a calm, reassuring voice. RL couldn't see the perspiration, the searching eyes, the tension and the concern I could see. Biochemistry is a vehicle for improvement, but sometimes someone has to care. ADA calls that the placebo effect. Scientific!

I don't ordinarily believe in testimonial letters, but I wanted to share this one with you:

Dear Dr. Huggins,

I have been through a living hell since I came down to see you. I came to see you on July 7, a month ago. When I went out to eat lunch, my left molars on the left side were so sore I could not chew. I was so mentally confused I had a hard time driving home. I could not chew for about two weeks and had to liquify all food in order to get some food. Dr. D-- was treating me for a viral infection, but Dr. C-- said I had a staph infection and an abcess on the lower left molar which he lanced. Dr. D-- started giving me antibiotic and a staph vaccine he uses. I was fatigued, mentally confused, fever went up over 100 (have never had that in my life). Dr. C-- started removing my silver fillings and gold cap. When he removed the lower left, that awful mental confusion I have had for years left immediately. I noticed it was easy to drive home. I could read my mail when I got home. I have never had that awful mental confusion since. He removed my last filling on July 22.

After I had the fillings removed, I was so extremely fatigued, depressed. BUT I COULD GO TO SLEEP. For years I had a hard time falling asleep, then would wake up, could not go back to sleep. But after those fillings were removed I ate breakfast, went back to sleep, got up for lunch, back to sleep, went to sleep after dinner. I slept night and day for over a week. I was so sick when I did wake up. Dr. D-- took me off the antibiotic. Said I was reacting to the antibiotic.

Am gradually getting stronger only need one nap a day.

GOD BLESS YOU

Abstracts For Your Enlightenment

The following abstracts of articles are presented for you to see some of the information which we have read and found to be important to our research efforts. There are many more articles than those presented here, but we feel that these will get you started toward an understanding of our position.

We are first presenting quotations from each article and then adding our comments which are found in italics.

Gastrointestinal and In Vitro Release of Copper, Cadmium, Indium, and Zinc from Conventional and Copper-rich Amalgam

C. Brune, et.al. published *Scand. J. Dent. Res.* 1983; 91:66-71

Particles of a conventional lathe-cut, a spherical non-gamma 2 and a copper amalgam have been gastrointestinally administered to rats for the purpose of evaluation of the dissolution resistance. The animals were sacrificed after 20 hours. The contents of copper, cadmium, indium, mercury and zinc in kidney, liver, lung and blood were measured using nuclear tracer techniques. From the copper amalgam an extreme release of copper was demonstrated. This study simulates the clinical condition of elemental fillings. Specimens of the same types of amalgams were also exposed to artificial saliva for a period of ten days. The amounts of copper and mercury released were measured with flame and flameless atomic absorption spectrophotometry respectively. The levels of copper and mercury released from the copper amalgam were approximately 50 times those of the two other amalgam types studied.

Comment:
This is an important article because it addresses two critical problems. First it shows that mercury does come out of amalgam, and second, it shows that the high copper amalgams release 50 TIMES MORE mercury than conventional amalgams. High copper amalgams are the most frequently placed amalgams today (1984). They are called "state of the art". Avoid them.

Allergy to Silver Amalgams

L.H. Catsakis published *Oral Surgery* 46:Sept 1978, 371-375

A patient with persistent periodontitis was cured when her silver amalgam restorations were replaced. She had a history of rash and swelling connected with wearing jewelry containing silver.

The patient was a 52-year-old woman who complained of severe periodontal problems which she said had begun seven years previously. Periodontal disease was evident and recent periodontal treatment had been ineffective. Clinical examination disclosed edematous gingival tissue that bled easily. Allergic reaction to the silver amalgam restorations was suspected, and the replacement of all of these was recommended. The patient decided to have only the four defective amalgam restorations on one side replaced. Soon after they were replaced with gold castings, the symptoms of periodontitis subsided on that side; the patient then decided to have the remaining restorations replaced. Meanwhile, patch tests confirmed the diagnosis. The response to silver nitrate 2 percent was blister formation and massive inflammation, followed by postinflammatory hyperpigmentation and scarring. Nickel sulfate 5 percent caused slight redness.

Shortly after the amalgam restorations were replaced, the periodontal tissues appeared healthy and remained so two years after treatment.

Comment:
This article shows the relationship between gum disease and the presence of silver mercury fillings. Removal of the fillings brought about healing of bleeding gums when conventional dental treatment did not help.

Hazards in Your Teeth

M. Hanson published *J. Orthomol. Psychiatry* Vol. 12, No. 3, Sept 1983

Glass vessels also absorb most of the mercury (Hg) from dilute solutions if precautions are not taken (Stock, 1939).

Comment:
This is the reason we use silicone baked linings in our urine sample tubes. This also explains why some scientific tests where urine was shipped overseas came out with zero results.

The vapor emission from silver amalgam is significant, also from old fillings. Stock (1939) measured levels of over 2 micrograms/M³ in respired air. At this level symptoms of poisoning appeared. The experiments have been repeated (Gay et al., 1979) and showed levels of 2.8 micrograms/M³ (14 ng/10 breaths) from one-week-old fillings and similar values from two year old fillings. After abrasion by chewing gum there was a sharp increase to 49 and 33 micrograms/M³ respectively. Further studies (Svare et al., 1981) showed that the levels were proportional to the number of fillings and values up to 87.5 micrograms/M³ were recorded. The authors also mention that the measured values probably were an underestimate. Mercury vaporizes fairly rapidly through centimeter-thick layers of water and saliva (Stock, 1939).

Comment:
These statements and studies address the question of mercury coming out of the fillings. They show that eating and gum chewing increase the amount of mercury released.

Till and Maly (1978) have recorded over 1200 micrograms/g tissue in the root of a tooth with both gold and amalgam and up to a few hundred micrograms/g in teeth with only amalgam.

Comment:
This study shows that the common practice of "amalgam build up" under gold crowns produces far more mercury in the bone and tissues around the tooth than just an amalgam filling alone. Keep in mind that they are not calling the "few hundred" micrograms safe. Others have shown that less than 10 micrograms can be damaging.

It is a metallurgical impossibility to find plastic amalgams which do not corrode and release mercury in the mouth.

Comment:
This says that the combination of metals in the mouth in conjunction with saliva will always produce a current. These are the essential ingre-

dients for a battery. This challenges the statements that say mercury cannot come out.

Stofen (1974) warns against the daily mercury load from amalgam and cites measurements by Stock (1939) of the amount of Hg in respired air and Radics et al (1970) of the loss of Hg from amalgam. In the latter study the amount of Hg, missing from an outer corroded zone (50-90 micrometers) was calculated to be up to 560 milligrams in a mouth with many fillings. If the loss has taken place during 10 years, the daily dose is 150 micrograms. Amalgam fillings can be very much more corroded than to a depth of 90 micrometers. Microphotos in a paper by Mateer and Reitz (1970) show corrosion in extracted fillings to a depth of at least 500 micrometers.

Comment:
There are many ideas of how much mercury constitutes a hazard. They range from 1 microgram to 100 micrograms. This study shows that this patient was possibly exposed to 150 micrograms from the fillings alone.

When one discusses the toxic effects of mercury from amalgam, one must consider that people are indiscriminately exposed: healthy and sick, strong and weak, children and adults, fertile and pregnant women. According to American gynecologists, fertile women should not be exposed to vapor levels higher than 10 micrograms/M^3 and pregnant women not to any raised levels at all (Koos and Longo, 1970). Hg vapor rapidly passes over to the unborn child and can cause damage, especially during the early phase of pregnancy. Hg is also excreted in milk during lactation. Female dentists and dental assistants are especially at risk. All types of mercury cause genetic damage (Verschaeve et all, 1976), are strongly immunotoxic (Koller, 1980) and induce antibiotic resistance in bacteria (Williams, 1971). Hg vapor which enters the nose (from amalgam during exhalation) passes rapidly to the brain and can be found in the olfactory lobe and tract, the pituitary gland and adjacent areas and has strong effect (Stock, 1935).

Comment:
This section points out an extremely important fact — some people are healthy and resistent — others are not. Mercury is always toxic. Fillings are placed indiscriminately. It also warns about placement of amalgam during pregnancy. The route from the filling to the brain may explain the origin of neurological diseases like multiple sclerosis, depression and epilepsy that respond to amalgam removal.

Mercury must be viewed as an extremely dangerous metal poison, especially considering its high vapor pressure, odorlessness, invisibility (as vapor) and long half-life in the brain; 18-22 years for the slowest component (Sugita, 1978).

Comment:
Another comment about mercury and brain tissue.

In a study on mercury in blood of mental patients, elevated levels were found in a number of cases especially among depressed patients and patients with several mental symptoms (Gowdy and Demers, 1978). There seems to be no reasonable source for the mercury other than the amalgam fillings since all patients lived under similar conditions. The authors consider 20 ng/g as a limit for normal levels. Levels over 7-8 ng/g indicate a recent significant exposure (Stock and Cucuel, 1934) and that was also the general level among the other mental patients.

Comment:
This statement relates depression and other mental disorders to the presence of silver-mercury fillings.

A comparison of the toxicity of different types of mercury shows that swallowed methylmercury and inhaled inorganic vapor are the most toxic forms and comparable in toxicity. The difference concerns mainly the distribution in various tissues. Both forms pass easily through membranes whereas ionized inorganic mercury sticks in membranes and there it coagulates proteins. Transport of necessary substances over the blood-brain barrier is disturbed and unspecific leakage is enhanced (Steinwall, 1968). A similar situation must exist in the placenta. Swallowed inorganic Hg-salts are absorbed to 15 percent with large individual variations (8-25 percent) (Rahoola et al, 1973): Methylmercury is almost completely absorbed in the intestines.

Comment:
This is almost a sleeper. When it mentions mercury sticking to the membranes and coagulating proteins, that is one of the most severe things it can do. Think of an egg as it fries. The albumin (protein) coagulates upon heating. Try to reverse that process. It also mentions that deadly methyl mercury "is almost completely absorbed in the intestines". Methyl mercury is what we hypothesize is the primary problem with amalgam fillings.

It is well known that metallic mercury in large drops generally can be swallowed without harm (obvious symptoms of poisoning). The absence of effects is just because it is in the form of large drops. However, deaths and severe poisonings have happened after swallowing metallic mercury. The larger the surface area, the more will be vaporized and absorbed.

Comment:
Very important concept. Vapor is the killer. Large puddles of mercury have small surface areas compared to vapor. Think of a teaspoon of water versus the amount of steam it can generate.

It is completely wrong to equate urinary excretion of Hg with the amount which has been given off from the amalgam, a fact which has been known for 50 years.

Comment:
Our big push in interpretation of urinary excretion of mercury links here. Our theory is that body excretion is related to body health more than to exposure.

Investigations during 1926-36 gave a very clear picture of mercury intoxication, both from amalgam and from industrial sources (Stock, 1936; Zangger, 1930; Fleischmann, 1928). The early symptoms of chronic mercurialism are largely subjective and mental: tiredness, "difficulty in getting up in the mornings", reduced energy and disposition for intellectual work, inner unrest (what we today would call type A behavior), depression, irritability, shyness, loss of memory (mainly short-term memory). Subsequently more objective somatic symptoms appear in chronic mercurialiasm: increased salivation, chronic catarrhs in the nose and upper airways, inflammations in the oral mucosa, easily bleeding gingiva, temporary loosening of teeth, "nervous heart", disturbed digestion, loss of appetite, sudden diarrheas, slight intestinal bleeding and pains, skin manifestations (eczema, dermatitis, urticaria), hearing difficulties, changes in vision (dim or double vision), speech and writing difficulties. Sudden changes in the condition without obvious reason is typical (Stock, 1926-39). Many additional symptoms were noted already by Stock and Fleischmann or have later been added: lymphocytosis, polyneuropathy, joint pains, sexual disturbances, fetal damage, thyroid changes, elevated cholesterol, increased caries frequency, elevated general susceptibility to disease and increased mortality (Stock, 1928; Fleischmann, 1928; Trachtenberg, 1974; Huggins, 1982). Individual variations are considerable. Each one is hit at his weakest point. The symptoms are very common in the civilized world but so are amalgam fillings. There is probably no other poison besides Hg which affects so many physiological processes.

Comment:
Everyone you read has a list of symptoms. Most overlap, but individual observers usually spot one or two symptoms no one else was looking for.

Current research shows that inorganic Hg is taken up by nerve endings and is transported towards the central nervous system (retrograde axonal transport).

Comment:
Another suggestion as to how multiple sclerosis, mental disturbances and epilepsy can show improvements after amalgam removal.

Blood Hg levels are only elevated after a recent, large exposure or after a long industrial exposure. The levels rapidly fall back to normal (5-8 ng/g) Stock and Cucuel, 1934; Cherian et al (1978). Blood tests as described by Huggins (1983) seem to be a better alternative.

Comment:
Our findings obviously agree. Blood mercury levels are corrected rapidly; have not proved to be an indicator of anything except large, recent exposures.

Composite plastics, being far from ideal, have in practice proved to be the best alternatives to amalgam. Adverse reactions are often caused by the mercury released from fillings, teeth and jawbone during the exchange. High carat gold is durable but will take up Hg from amalgam fillings if both metals are simultaneously present in the mouth, also without contact with each other (Stock, 1928). They might also take up Hg from the saliva which is a secretion pathway for Hg (Joselow and Goldwater, 1968).

Comment:
The hidden meaning here is that amalgam and gold do not belong together in the same mouth. Electrochemical reactions increase. We have noted in our practice that many people tolerate amalgam with a minimum of difficulty until a gold crown is placed, then BOOM! This last

straw breaks the patient's resistance and multiple symptoms emerge rapidly.

Allergy to mercury is often not testable on the skin. A patch test might show nothing at the application site but eczema can flare up at another part of the body. Immune reactions in the blood are the first reactions after exposure to mercury (Trachktenberg, 1974; Huggins, 1982). A person can be extremely sensitive to inhaled Hg without showing a positive skin reaction (Stock, 1936).

Comment:
Patch testing is a screening test, but as this statement reflects, what we are looking for is a physiological, systemic reaction. Skin reactions are a very small part of the diagnosis.

The majority of people might have sufficient resistance to Hg to have amalgam without becoming seriously ill. However, mercury kills cells which are not renewed, especially nerve cells. These cells are the ones we will need later in life as a reserve. No dentist can guarantee that the patient will not come to harm.

Comment:
I am reminded of the fellow who said, "If I had known I was going to live this long I would have taken better care of myself." Mercury damages cells daily. At some point in time we run out of reserve healthy cells and sickness results. Many people have high resistance in youth, but what about when you get older, say 35 and above?

Organotin compounds are extremely toxic. Silver causes argyria, an irreversible gray discoloration of the skin. The possibility of "inner argyria" has not been investigated. Silver binds extremely strongly to proteins and is used in the most sensitive protein stain available and also to stain nerve cells.

Comment:
We have cautioned a great deal about mercury, but we should also keep in mind that mercury is not the only element coming out of the filling. On the scale of most reactive, tin is the "least noble" of the metals in an amalgam, therefore it should leach out first. This quote shows that tin and silver both cause toxic problems on their own. This is in addition to what mercury is doing.

Mercury Poisoning from Dental Amalgam

J. Pleva published *J. Orthomol. Psych.* Vol. 12, No. 3. Sept. 1983.

Analyses of saved silver amalgam fillings showed that they were badly corroded. Corrosion attacks on almost every aged amalgam filling show that assurances that amalgam is a stable alloy can be dismissed. Statements that amalgam is not harmful are unfounded and based on short-term considerations. Galvanic coupling of gold and amalgam gives a guarantee for mercury poisoning within a relatively short time. The label "oral galvanism" is insufficient and misleading since the problem is crevice corrosion of amalgam.

The dangers of insidious mercury intoxication from amalgam are known at least since the 1920s, but after more than half a century the problem seems more to the fore than ever. Voices have often been raised, warning that silver amalgam (and before that copper amalgam) is not harmless and describing symptoms of poisoning. In spite of this, the amalgam situation in the mouth is seldom considered in medical practice. A study of the subject and today's situation, leads one to conclude that the dental and medical care systems have serious deficiencies in knowledge of important border sciences like corrosion chemistry and toxicology.

Comment:
This author has a doctorate in corrosion chemistry. Corrosion is the action of metallic breakdown we are seeing in fillings. His reaction is that of a chemist who himself was poisoned by amalgam. His major thrust is to make dentists (who use metals but have no training in metallurgy) aware of the electrochemical problems they are producing in the body.

A state of indescribable tiredness, stress and anxiety was constantly present. To perform simple tasks, to join discussions, to think, talk and to be social required considerable effort. During visits to doctors I mainly complained about my irregular heart. Since all tests were in general normal (a slightly elevated cholesterol level), the patient imagines his troubles. To several doctors I pointed out that there was an amalgam filling in the gold bridge, a filling which after a few months had become black and rough which indicated corrosion and dissolution of the amalgam. No doctor was interested in this fact.

Comment:
Historically this is what got the chemist Pleva interested in studying mercury toxicity.

SYMPTOMS OF THE AMALGAM SYNDROME

Irregular heartbeat, often together with anxiety
Strong pains in the left part of the chest
Retinal bleeding
Dim vision, especially after exercise; slow and poor accommodation
Inability to fix gaze, uncontrollable eye movements. Eyes drawing to one side.
Geometric figures in the visual field, migrating in a few minutes from the periphery towards the center and slowly disappearing.
A "film" over the eyes, dry eyes
Arcus senilis: a grey ring around the cornea (permanent)
Red irritated throat; inflammation in upper airways and pleurisy a year after the dental treatment.
Difficulties in swallowing
Severe amnesia; constant strain; anxiety; irritability; difficulty and even impossibility to control behavior; indecision
Loss of interest in life; tiredness; a feeling of being old
Resistance to intellectual work; reduced capacity for work, both intellectual and physical; reduced powers of comprehension, information does not come through
Increased need for sleep
Vertigo
Headache (about once a week), often migraine-like, especially induced by weather changes and by prolonged sleep in the mornings
Facial paralysis, right side and partly permanent. Damage to balance and hearing
A painful pull at the lower jaw towards the collar bone
Increased salivation, sour metallic taste
Bleeding gums at toothbrushing
Joint pains, especially increasing 1981-2
Pains in the lower back
Weakness of muscles, slow muscle action
Pressure, pains, "needles" in the liver region
Asthmatic breathing troubles, a feeling of not being able to breathe, "cracking" in the lower part of the pleural sac, forcing to cough
Gastrointestinal irritation
"Needles" at lymph nodes under arms and in groin
Eczema

Comment:
This is a cumulative list of symptoms that overcame Dr. Pleva while becoming mercury toxic from his fillings. Over a period of months after

amalgam removal, all symptoms reversed to normal. The last to return to normal was the facial paralysis.

Since no doctor could help me I tried to find the cause by myself. I noticed that the surface of the amalgam filling (about 4x4mm) in the gold bridge (surface 670 mm²) rather quickly became black and rugged. As a corrosion specialist I was fully aware of the fact that this was a galvanic cell where the more noble gold was the cathode and the amalgam the anode. This meant that the anode/amalgam was dissolving and that the metal ionized as cations.

Comment:
Dr. Pleva's thinking as he was forced to diagnose and treat his own disease.

When the fillings opposite the gold bridge were removed, every tendency to headache or migraine disappeared. the change was so abrupt I can see no other explanation than the removal of the fillings in these still living teeth. In writing this, headache has not reappeared except once, after a dental treatment when several fillings were drilled out and presumably some amalgam was swallowed and inhaled.

Comment:
Again, reference to the incredible reactions that occur when amalgams and gold are placed in the same mouth.

When all fillings had been removed, all symptoms except the facial paralysis and arcus senilis rather quickly diminished in about three months. Subjectively the mental abilities and memory seemed to recover more slowly than the somatic functions. However, mental functions are more difficult to quantify than symptoms of more physical character, for example irregular heart and difficulties in breathing.

Some symptoms I had thought to have other causes than amalgam also disappeared, especially back ache, which I related to office work and my height (190 cm). Also the pains below the ribs which were thought to be remnants of a hepatitis 20 years earlier, disappeared. In December 1982 I also found that small vesicles and exfoliation of the epidermis on the sole of one foot and on the insides of my hands completely disappeared.

Comment:
Description of the healing process that occurred as a result of amalgam removal.

The improvements in my health could not be related to any factor in my surroundings: work, home, personal relations or diet since these remained unchanged. The disappearance of the symptoms clearly falls into the period of amalgam removal and afterwards. Finally I want to stress the amazing improvement in well-being, only three months after the final dental treatment. In spite of still improving, I have regained a feeling of peace and calmness, of being able to appreciate smells, details and gradations in my surroundings, something I must go back 10-15 years to find. I no longer accept that a 40-year-old person must have some age-related symptoms: tiredness, headache or pains in some places. According to my opinion, a prerequisite for health is that corroding alloys, releasing highly toxic heavy metals, are removed from the oral cavity.

Comment:
This is in defense against those people who will say that what occurred was a spontaneous remission, or that something unreported was the reason for symptom remission.

Some pieces of amalgam fillings, removed in 1982, have been saved and analyzed for corrosion attacks and composition with a JEOL scanning electron microscope with EDAX (Energy Dispersive Analysis with X-Rays) equipment. The first apparent features, visible with the naked eye, both on these and other fillings, were that their surfaces towards the tooth cavities, were largely black. Fig. 1 [in his original article] shows an example of corrosion at the margin of a filling (five years old). The surfaces were clearly corroded, most severely near the margins towards the outer electrolyte (saliva), a feature which is characteristic for crevice cell corrosion.

A selective dissolution of the least corrosion resistant phase in the metallographically complex amalgam system has been observed many times and has been accepted as one of the most common causes for corrosion of silver amalgam (Jorgensen, 1965; Guthrow et al., 1967; Sarkar et al., 1975). Corrosion of this phase releases metallic mercury which can either ionize, evaporate or partly react with the other phases to form [a] new corrodible phase and the attack can continue (Espevik, 1977). The filling becomes porous which enhances corrosion and causes the margins to crack (Fig 1., Jorgensen, 1975). Severe corrosion could be seen, not only between filling and tooth, but also on the free surface towards the cheek.

Surfaces and the inner of fillings were analyzed with the EDAX equipment. The inner surface of the fillings showed no considerable difference between the two silver amalgam fillings aged 5 and 20 years. The mercury content of 40 percent was lower than in freshly prepared amalgam which contained 45 percent mercury. The new amalgam contained significantly higher amounts of copper relative to the silver content, which suggests a new type of amalgam. From the chemical and electrochemical point of view, the increased copper content (14 percent) must be considered completely unsuitable since copper is easily dissolved to easily soluble compounds (Wrangen & Berendson, 1982).

Analyses of the black corrosion products in the crevices yeilded interesting information. The smooth black surface of a five year old filling contained 27 percent mercury, 3 percent silver and 66 percent tin. The black, porous surfaces of a 20 year old filling were devoid of mercury and silver and contained 40-60 percent tin, 37-51 percent zinc and 4-7 percent copper.

Comment:
This is a very important disclosure scientifically. As a corrosion chemist, he put his primary skills to work proving that mercury and other metals do leach out of amalgams.

It is a well known fact that amalgam of every known composition corrodes (Schoonover and Souder, 1941; Mateer and Reitz, 1970).

Comment:
Again, substantiation that amalgam is chemically reactive in the oral environment.

I have observed my surroundings and questioned about 150 people with symptoms similar to those I experienced myself. A causal relation between their troubles and their dental status seems to emerge. The relation is most clearly seen when there are gold restorations which can come into contact with amalgam, but also when there are many large amalgam fillings and no gold. It is remarkable that no broad investigation on these relations has been carried out already a long time ago, for instance within the scope of investigations on the etiology of civilization diseases.

Comment:
This addresses several common questions. How many people are sensitive? Dr. Pleva had no trouble in finding 150 people. He also addresses the subject of gold and amalgam together in the same mouth. The really important question, and the one no one wants to answer is directed to the observation, "no broad investigation has been carried out."

It has recently been shown that mercury, in the same amounts as those released from amalgam (estimated), can produce periodontitis in germ-free animals (Till, 1978).

Comment:
Now we have reference to amalgam-related gum disease in both humans and animals.

Corrosion will lead to an enrichment of mercury in the surface layer, an increase in partial pressure and a subsequent higher level in the vapor phase.

Measurements on extracted teeth have shown that mercury migrates from amalgam fillings to root and jaw bone and can be enriched there. When there has been contact with gold, the level can reach more than 1200 ppm (parts/million, micrograms/gram tissue), (Till and Maly, 1978).

Mercury is released from amalgam in the mouth in considerable amounts through various mechanisms. These can be enhanced by mechanical, thermal, electrolytic and bacterial factors (Wagner and Till, 1973; Wagner and Till, 1974; Till, 1977, Wranglen and Berendson, 1982).

The term "oral galvanism" is misleading since the main problem is corrosion and release of toxic metals.

Reports on corrosion of amalgam, published by dental institutions, often indicate a misunderstanding of possible corrosion mechanisms (Nilner, 1981; Glantz and Bergman, 1982); such questions should be handled by competent technical institutions. Sweeping, unfounded statements like "passivation of the surface of metallic dental materials is a commonly occurring phenomenon which means that the intraoral corrosion can be so insignificant that it can practically be considered to have ceased" (Glantz and Bergman, 1982) cannot be considered sufficient justification for loading the mouth with grams of mercury, often in combination with gold.

The statement that there have never been reports on systematic dissolution of silver amalgam fillings (Glantz and Bergman, 1982) has no foundation in reality. Almost any old amalgam filling, viewed through the microscope, shows attack by crevice corrosion. Disregarding the questions of the stability of single restorations, it is primarily the very common and thoughtless use of combinations of metals like gold and amalgam which indicates that dentists today have little qualification to prevent poisoning of their patients. More education and interest are needed to take advantage of present knowledge.

For the same reasons, statements that there are no reasons to advise dentists against the use of amalgam and that people should not be imparted the belief that we face considerable health problems (Friberg, 1982), do not reflect the real situation and are worthless when it comes to solving existing problems.

Comment:
All these sections exphasize the age old question about whether mercury can get out of a filling or not. He somewhat chastises the health professions for their oblivion to current knowledge on metal chemistry.

Similarly, when the amalgam fillings in the right part of the lower jaw were removed, the painful strain after the facial paralysis, present four years, disappeared. It seems close at hand to suspect a combination of the general poisoning and the mercury source in the two teeth in the lower jaw as primary causes of the nerve inflammation, resulting in the face paralysis on the same side.

Comment:
The facial paralysis was the last symptom to respond. I am sure he wonders, as we do, how many paralyses are there today that could go away after amalgam removal?

The correct approach is not first to use amalgam and then to demand that the patient himself shall prove that amalgam caused the ensuing problems. First it must be proved that amalgam is not harmful and that it does not corrode.

Comment:
Another chastisement to the health scientific community. Why make the patient prove the material is harmful? Isn't that the responsibility of the professions?

Epidemiology, Etiology, and Prevention of Multiple Sclerosis

T.H. Ingalls, *J. Forensic Med. and Path.*, Vol. 4, No. 1. March 1983.

Slow retrograde seepage of ionic mercury from root canal or Class V amalgam fillings inserted many years previously, recurrent caries and corrosion around filling edges, and the oxidizing effect of the purulent response may lead to multiple sclerosis in middle age. Epidemiologic studies of MS consistently reveal less neurological disease in the south, inferentially because there may be less caries and therefore fewer fillings done in the south. Clinical and epidemiologic data also suggest that a second heavy metal, lead, may operate almost interchangeably with mercury. Possibly, cases of unilateral MS derived from mercury amalgam fillings in ipsilateral teeth, whereas the generalized disease may result from ingestion or inhalation of volatile mercury or exhaust fumes of lead additives to gasoline. The forensic and preventive medical challenge is to identify, monitor, and resolve questions of hidden heavy metal hazards in a high technology society, especially those of lead and mercury. Further clinical epidemiologic and basic science studies of heavy metal assays in whole blood, CNS tissues, packed cells, and serum are warranted. Prevention awaits further testing of the hypothesis and experience with substitute filling materials.

Comment:
Dr. Ingalls, an MD with multiple credentials has multiple sclerosis himself. He related retrograde amalgams (amalgam fillings at the root tip of some root canal treated teeth), the amalgam filling and lead as sources that can cause neurologic disturbances resulting in what is called multiple sclerosis.

Methylation of Mercury from Dental Amalgam and Mercuric Chloride by Oral Streptococci In Vitro.

Ulf. Heintze published *Scand. J. Dent. Res.* 1983.; 91; 150-2

The capacity of the oral bacteria *Streptococcus mitior*, *S. mutans*, and *S. sanguis* to methylate mercury was investigated *in vitro*. Mercuric chloride and pulverized dental amalgam in distilled water, respectively, were used as sources of mercury. Methyl mercury was found in the bacterial cells of all three tested strains. The results indicate that organic mercury compounds may be formed in the oral cavity.

The biologic methylation of mercury can follow alternative pathways and may either be totally abiotic, i.e., without intervention of microbes, or the result of a microbial metabolism.

The results indicate the possibility of a microbial methylation of inorganic mercury from amalgam restorations in the mouth, as the oral streptococci studied are common in the dental plaque. *S. mitior* is also found in large numbers on the mucous membranes of the oral cavity.

Several strains of bacteria and yeasts are capable of degrading methyl mercury to inorganic mercury.

In the present study, the release of mercury from both conventional and non gamma-2 amalgam was comparable which is in agreement with the findings of Brune.

Methyl mercury was found in the bacterial cells of all four tested strains when they had grown in the presence of mercury chloride or corrosion products of amalgam. When cultured in the mercury chloride broth, the concentration of methyl mercury was larger with the streptococcal strains than with *Clostridium cochlearium T-2* (the control species). No methyl mercury was detected in the supernatant fluids.

Comment:
This is one of the most important articles we have found. It's significance is in the fact that Streptococcus mutans, and S. mitiore both live in everyone's mouth, and that they can manufacture methyl mercury. Deadly methyl mercury is 100 TIMES more toxic to the nervous system than plain elemental mercury. This could really help explain multiple sclerosis, epilepsy and a multitude of neural as well as emotional disturbances.

The mention of yeast brings to mind the connection we see between methyl mercury and *Candida Albicans.*

Since more methyl mercury was produced by *Strep mutans* than by the control methyl producer, one could conclude that significant quantities could be produced right on the filling surface.

Methyl Mercury Poisoning in Fish and Human Beings.

T.B. Eyl, published *Mod. Med.,* Vol. 38., Nov. 16, 1970.

It was not generally known that the relatively inoffensive metal is converted, before entering the algae-fish-human food chain, into one of the most potent and insidious poisons in existence, namely, *organic* methyl mercury. This biological methylation is accomplished by bacteria called *Methanobacterium omelanskii* living in the bottom mud. These bacteria are then eaten by plankton, which in turn are eaten by fish. Contaminated species include pike, pickerel, perch, walleye, muskie, and white bass. Methylation is carried out under mostly anaerobic conditions and is facilitated by the presence of raw sewage discharged into the water by industrial and municipal sources.

Methyl mercury, unlike inorganic Hg compounds, is an extremely subtle, difficult-to-detect, and long lasting poison. It is bound by hemoglobin in the red blood cells and circulates in this form for months, being excreted at the rate of only 1 percent per day, mostly in the feces; the estimated half-life in man is seventy days and in fish two hundred days. It passes easily into the central nervous system, where it selectively and irreversibly damages the cells of the granular layer in the cerebellum, the cerebral cortex, and the calcarine cortex. It swiftly passes the placental barrier and accumulates in the fetal brain and blood, building up to 30 percent higher red blood cell levels than in the mother. It appears, further, to be more cumulative in female than in male blood and to be *especially injurious* to the central nervous system of infants and children.

Comment:
If methyl mercury is a problem from fillings, then we should be aware of the additional amount from sea foods. It does add up.

Intensive investigations of Hg levels in wild fowl, fish, and human beings also have been carried out in Canada. In March of this year, the Canadian government informed U.S. authorities that fish caught in the Great Lakes and adjacent waters had Hg (virtually 100 percent methyl mercury) levels up to 2.8 ppm. More recently, levels up to 9 ppm have been found in a few specimens. A chemical plant in Sarnia, Ontario, was estimated to be discharging up to 200 lb. of "waste" metallic Hg daily into the St. Clair River, which flows between Lake Huron and Lake Erie.

Comment:
There are reports that the mercury level is coming down, but to clean out trillions of gallons of water and bacteria laden mud in a lake that size would seem like a multicentury task.

Many scientists recommend, for safety, that a whole blood level of approximately 100 ppb should not be exceeded. This would correspond to a daily intake of 0.1 mg of Hg, or about 100 gm of fish containing 1 ppb (mg/kg) of Hg.

Comment:
This is the highest toxic factor we have found. Toxic ranges run from 1 to 100 parts per billion. It does make one stop and think about just how much fish should be consumed. Perhaps we should just give up eating. No, but it is well to know how much exposure we are subjected to and very helpful to know how to partly compensate for the exposures.

Professor Tejning of the University of Lund, Sweden, has demonstrated in five instances that fetal red blood cells at birth contained an average concentration of Hg 28 percent higher than that of the mother. Moreover, the higher the maternal red blood cell level, the faster the rate of increase in fetal red blood cell Hg levels; in other words, the rise in fetal red blood cell levels is disproportionately rapid at the higher maternal levels. The accentuated effects of methyl mercury on the fetus are attested by the fact that in nineteen Minamata cases of infantile cerebral paresis the mothers showed no typical clinical symptoms of poisoning, except for some complaints of numbness during pregnancy, although they were all heavy fish-eaters. On the basis of these facts it must be recommended, pending further studies, that pregnant women abstain from eating fish contaminated with methyl mercury.

The second question, about which we know even less, is that of the effects of methyl mercury on genetics. Swedish Prof. Claes Ramel has shown that methyl mercury is 1,000 times more potent in causing genetic damage than the next most powerful agent known — colchicine.

Comment:
This information is of value to the pregnant female. More and more data is accumulating that implies, don't expose your unborn baby to mercury. Our biggest concern is that mercury is not excreted well in people suffering from mercury toxicity. Another point of interest in pregnancy is Ramels comment that methyl mercury is extremely potent in the area of genetic damage. If negative current fillings are responsible for greater methyl mercury formation, then the new high copper amalgams that so frequently register negative current certainly would not be desirable during pregnancy.

Reaction of the Human Dental Pulp to Silver Amalgam Restorations

B. Moller published *Swed. Dent. J.,* Vol. 2, 1978, 93-97.

In cell culture studies, newly prepared amalgam had an immediate and marked cytotoxic effect comparable to that of mercury.

Comment:
Note how this directly contradicts material presented by the ADA at their news conference July 13, 1984. "When mercury is combined with the metals used in dental amalgam, its toxic properties are made harmless."

Mercury Content in Gingival Tissues Adjacent to Amalgam Fillings.

H. Freden, et.al. published *Odont. Revy.* 25, 1974, 207-210.

All amalgam restorations were older than three years. All the (tissue) biopsies which had been in contact with amalgam restorations showed markedly higher mercury contents than did the control biopsies. . . . a high of 380 micrograms per gram of tissue was found in test biopsies, and a high of only 10 micrograms per gram of tissue was found in the control biopsies.

Comment:
This study shows that not only does mercury come out of the fillings, but that the amount recorded in the gum tissues is far greater close to amalgam than in non-amalgam exposed tissue.

Corrosion of Gold and Amalgam Placed in Contact with Each Other.

T. Fusayama, et.al. published *J. Dent. Res.* 1963, 42, 1183-1197.

Schoonover and Souder have reported that gold restorations were corroded by mercury released from amalgam fillings because of an electrochemical reaction. Since then, most dental textbooks have recommended against the use of gold in contact with amalgam in the mouth. It is a fact, however, that many dental clinicians are routinely using them in contact with each other.

Comment:
It is interesting to note that even though this statement appears to be mentioned in textbooks, no one lecturing on crown and bridge techniques mentions it in seminars. It is a virtually unknown and undiscussed topic among dentists.

The Mechanism of Marginal Fracture of Amalgam Fillings

K.D. Jorgensen published *JADA,* Vol. 28, 1941, 1278-91.

Due to the corrosion of the amalgam margin, metallic mercury is set free. The loss of substance can also be observed on polished sections of amalgam margins: porosities which is an evident consequence of corrosion occur here especially in the part of the amalgam facing the cavity walls.

Comparative Epidemiology of Multiple Sclerosis and Dental Caries.

W. Craelium published *J. Epidemiology and Community Health,* 1978, 32, 155-165.

Multiple sclerosis is virtually unknown in the tropics, and numerous studies and reviews have documented that living in sunny climates, especially during the very early years of life offers one protection against acquiring MS. Certain populations, however, like the Eskimos, appear to be protected against acquiring MS in spite of their extremely low sunlight exposures.

Dental caries has been recently added to the WHO compilation and this disease is here reported to share many epidemiological features in common with MS. Casual comparison of the WHO map of dental caries incidences throughout the world reveals a striking parallel in general trend.

Comparison of DMF teeth with the MS death rates results in a correlation coefficient of 0.97, and the probability of a chance occurence is less than 0.002. This represents a nearly perfect linear relationship between dental disease rates and MS death rates.

It has been suggested that the DMF index may vary directly with the level of care, because dentists tend to fill undecayed teeth as a prophylactic measure.

An extremely low or zero rate of MS was reported among the Eskimos in the area around Anchorage, Alaska during the period 1950 to 1963. This correlates with the very low rate of caries found among Eskimos from the same area in a survey in 1960.

Another important test case not included in the correlation is that of the 15 million Bantus of South Africa, who are possibly unique in the total absence among them of any reported MS cases. Dental surveys in 1937 and more recently in 1975 have found extremely low rates of caries among this population. Sixty percent of rural Bantus ages 16 to 17 years were entirely free from caries and 33 percent of urban Bantus. The average DMF for both rural and urban Bantus was 1.7. These figures are among the lowest found anywhere in the world.

The first report on MS among non-whites in South Africa has recently appeared. The cases included seven colored people and one Indian. The appearance of MS for the first time among these racial groups is interesting in view of their declining dental health. Among the English speaking white population, the prevalence of MS was 11 per 100,000 in a survey in 1960, but since 1964 there have been well documented annual increases in new cases of MS among the whites, and current prevalence is certainly higher. An increasing frequency of dental caries in this population was noted 20 years before the increase in MS.

The highest frequency of MS is found in Northern Ireland and the Scottish islands, and these areas of the world also rank highest in dental disease.

A study of Orientals living in California and Washington indicated that this group had a much lower risk of MS than Causasians. Parallel results are found for dental disease. Chinese residents of the United States were found to have the lowest rate of DMF teeth of any ethnic group examined in a large military study.

MS is generally more common in women than in men, and dental caries are more prevalent in women of all age groups than in men, according to national surveys in the U.S., Iceland, England, Scotland, Germany, and Polynesia.

Pregnancy and lactation increase the risk of MS and of dental caries too.

MS in Northern Ireland is significantly more frequent among agricultural workers compared with employers, managers, and professionals. Apparently opposite to the trend in the U.S. dental disease follows the MS pattern in Northern Ireland; a recent survey found significantly more dental caries among manual compared with non-manual workers.

The search for an MS virus has so far proved fruitless; it is interesting to consider the possibility that the etiologies of dental caries and MS are similar.

The possibility that the close correlations found between MS and dental disease are due to chance is extremely unlikely, and it has been shown that MS prevalence varies with actual rates of dental disease and not simply with dental indices which are influenced by levels of dental care. Increases in the prevalence of dental caries both in South Africa and in the Scottish islands have been followed by increases in the prevalence of MS.

Comment:

All of these references point up a relationship between cavities and multiple sclerosis. Taking this hypothesis one step further, we feel that there is substantial evidence for a link to those cavities being filled with amalgam. If not, why do so many cases of MS improve when amalgam is removed sequentially?

The National Multiple Sclerosis Society in conjunction with the American Dental Association does not share this feeling. The NMSS sent a letter on April 1, 1983 to all chapters. We received a copy from them in May of 1984. Why the delay we don't know. They recommended that patients with MS keep their amalgams. We wrote to Robert J. Slater, MD (medical director) explaining that we had seen improvements after sequential removal of amalgam. We asked him to respond — nothing. We are frequently asked why we don't inform the MS society of our findings. We have on several occasions and either get referred to a dentist on staff who "never heard of such a thing", or does as Slater did — nothing. Why?

Mercury

L.W. Chang published in *Experimental and Clinical Neurotoxicity*

Among all the mercury compounds, alkyl mercury, particularly methyl mercury is found to be most neurotoxic.

Experimental studies indicated that over 90 percent of ingested methyl mercury was rapidly absorbed. Studies on human volunteers also indicated an almost complete absorption of methyl mercury salt.

In short-chain alkylmercury compounds, e.g. methyl mercury, mercury penetrates the erythrocyte membrane and binds to hemoglobin. Such binding is reversed by providing extracellular sulfhydryl groups. The binding of methyl mercury to erythrocytes is tighter in rats than in humans. No difference in stability in binding was observed between adult and fetal erythrocytes. (Comment: *Erythrocytes are red blood cells.*)

"Biotransformation" may be referred to as the changes of oxidative state of the mercury, or the formation and cleavage of covalent bonds of the organic mercurials in the biological system. Mercury vapor is readily oxidized to mercuric ion in blood and tissue. Catalase is considered to be the enzyme responsible for the oxidation of elemental mercury.

A study by Syverson indicates that more inorganic mercury is retained in the brain after injection of methyl mercury than after an equal dose of mercuric chloride.

Although all mercuric compounds should be considered systemic toxicants, the critical organ for inorganic mercury (e.g. mercuric chloride) is the kidney, and for alkyl mercury (e.g. methyl mercury) is the nervous system.

It is obvious that mercury compounds, either organic or inorganic in nature, exert their toxic effects in a generalized systemic manner. Thus, besides the nervous system, other organ systems such as liver, kidney, or endocrine glands are also affected by the toxic metal to a certain extent. Moreover, the overall pathological impacts of mercury upon adult systems and upon fetal systems are drastically different.

Most of the patients with neurological problems attributable to inorganic mercury intoxication have been victims of occupational exposures. Among all possible routes of exposure, dust inhalation is probably the most common and frequent, with ingestion following very closely. Ingestion is more usual among workers who have contaminated their hands or fingers with mercury compounds. Depending on the frequency and dose of exposure, the onset of symptoms of inorganic mercury poisoning may be delayed as long as 30 years.

With respect to the uptake of inorganic mercury in the brain, it was found that the total was several times greater in vapor-exposed animals than in injected animals.

Unlike the heterogeneous distribution seen in the case of inorganic mercury, the distribution of the methyl mercuric salt was more uniform. The areas showing maximum concentration of mercury were the hippocampus and the cerebellar gray matter. However, Yoshino and co-workers demonstrated that in dogs the calcarine cortex and the cerebellum showed higher mercury levels. A recent study by Semjen and associates also found that after subchronic, continuous administration of radioactive labeled methyl mercuric hydroxide to rats, the spinal dorsal root ganglia contained the highest concentration of mercury, followed closely by the cerebral cortex and the cerebellum, then the subcortical part of the forebrain.

Occupational Exposure to Mercury

L.J. Goldwater published *Arch Environ Health.* Vol. 17, July 1968

In the dental group, on the other hand, about 90 percent of the population did show mercury in their urine in amounts that ranged from 10 micrograms to 155 micrograms per liter. That dentists as a group are absorbing mercury is clearly indicated by these data.

Comment:
This article clearly shows that dentists are exposed to mercury at levels that should be addressed. Dentists as a whole are not made aware of their personal hazard, nor of the hazard to the patient. Data like this should at least make the dentist conscious of a need for his own personal safety. Hopefully someday that courtesy will be extended to his patients as well.

Mercury Contamination in the Dental Office.

V.W. Rinne published *J. Nebr. Dent. Assoc.*

The study was undertaken because dental students were being taught to wring out the excess mercury from the silver alloy mercury mixture and the excess mercury eventually landed on the clinic floor. The magnitude of the problem became obvious when it was determined that 21 pounds of mercury had been dispensed during the 1966-67 school year. The ratio of mercury to silver alloy which was used at that time was eight to five so it could be assumed that eight pounds of mercury had been expressed and deposited as a contaminant during a one year period. If, as assumed, eight pounds of mercury had been deposited in one year, then a much larger amount of free mercury would be present in the clinic as a result of accumulations during the previous forty years.

The report revealed that fingernails from 13 individuals in this group contained mercury well above what could be considered to be safe. The range varied from 5.5 ppm (parts per million) to 252 ppm. Although it is difficult to state exactly what amount of mercury found in fingernails would be considered to be harmful, the average for the United States is from 5 to 6 ppm. It would be safe to conclude then, that any amount above ten ppm could be considered to be well above normal limits.

At the end of the 1967 summer session the College of Dentistry began the move to a new building on the East Campus. During the period of August through October, school was not in session and dental students and assistants were not exposed to mercury vapor.

The second sample of fingernail clippings was taken in November 1967 before the students and assistants started work in the clinic. This sample included 18 dental students and assistants. There was only one individual in this group whose analysis was reported to be above the 10 ppm limit. The range was from 0.259 ppm. to 14.9 ppm.

Comment from HAH:
This report on clinical contamination bothers me somewhat, because that was the dental school I attended.

More About Mercury Hygiene

H. Buchwald published *Canadian For. Dent. Services.* Vol. 12, Oct. 1971.

Dental assistants generally prepared the amalgam and accumulated significant amounts of residual mercury on their hands. Swab samples from assistants' hands in some cases contained more than 1 mg of mercury. Microscopic examination of the hands showed the mercury to be in the form of tiny droplets capable of lodging in pores and fissures. Finely divided mercury in this form may eventually dissolve and be absorbed through the skin; alternatively it may be transferred to food, cigarettes or directly into the mouth. Such mercury from the mouth or in food will dissolve in gastric juices and be absorbed. Mercury on cigarettes, collected from contaminated hands or working surfaces will inevitably be vaporized and inhaled. It was observed that dental assistants were not always careful to wash their hands after using mercury and between patients.

Of 23 dentists interviewed only 11 were aware that mercury could be harmful but only two took any precautions in using mercury. Out of 25 assistants only seven were aware that mercury could be harmful.

Comment:
With responses of "noninformed" from active professionals in dentistry, is it any wonder that the lay person has no concept of mercury toxicity? Most lay people are not even aware that silver fillings contain mercury, much less know that they contain 50 percent mercury.

Mercury Vapor Exposure in Dental Offices

P.A. Gronka, et.al. published *JADA* 81: 23-925 Oct. 1970.

Many homes of dentists may have high levels of mercury contamination caused by the dentist's carrying mercury metal into the home by contaminated shoes.

Editorial, *JADA*, Vol. 82, March 1971.

Are amalgam fillings and their placement hazardous to the patient? The answer is an unqualified "NO". Study after study has shown that the patient undertakes no risk whatsoever with the amalgam filling.

His encounter with mercury vapor during insertion of the filling is too brief and the total amount of mercury vapor involved is too small. Neither would the ingestion of a portion of the filling material place him in jeopardy. Again, his encounter with mercury would be too brief and the total amount involved too small.

Comment:
It is interesting to note that there is no documentation to this "study after study" claim. Efforts to find these studies proved fruitless. We contacted Dr. P.L. Fan of the ADA to request reprints of those studies. He said he would be happy to furnish them. A few days later we received one reprint (written before we were born) and a list of references that, in his words, "clearly repudiate any apprehension about the safety of amalgam fillings." In case you missed them in the body of the book, we shall repeat some of the more apprehension repudiating titles:

"Death Caused by Swallowing Large Amalgam Filling"
"Diseased Eyes and Amalgam Fillings"
"Mercurial Necrosis Resulting from Amalgam Fillings"
"A Shameful Case of Malpractice (Amalgam Filling)"
"Irritation of the Larynx Caused by an Amalgam Filling"
"Poisoning from Corrosive Sublimate Generated in the Mouth from Amalgam Plugs in the Teeth"
"A Consideration of the Objections Offered by Physicians to Amalgam Fillings"
"Mercurial Poisoning and Amalgam Fillings"
"Case of Deafness Probably Caused by Amalgam Fillings"
"Injurious Effects of Amalgam"
"Salivation Produced by Mixing Amalgams in the Hand"
"The Itinerant Amalgam Peddlers"
"Amalgam and Kindred Poisons"
"In View of the Recent Investigations, Has Amalgam Been a Blessing or Curse to Humanity?"
"Oral Electricity and the New Departure (Amalgam)"
"Amalgam Filling Causing Acid Taste"
"The Amalgam Fraud"
"Death From an Amalgam Plug"
"Acute Mania Attributed to an Amalgam Filling"
"The Amalgam Question Again — Its Moral Aspect"
"The Poisonous Effects of Amalgam Fillings"

Handling of Mercury,

C.W. Mayhall, C.J. Andres published *JADA* 82: 1271, June 1971.

Fresh amalgam continues to release mercury vapor for several minutes after mixing. This source may also be eliminated by storing amalgam scraps under water as soon as they are no longer needed.

Summary of the International Conference on Mercury Hazards in Dental Practice

P. Bloch, I.M. Shapiro published *JADA* Vol 104, April 1982.

Knowledge of the toxicity of mercury should be a mandatory part of the training of dental students and all other dental personnel who come in contact with mercury.

Mercury Toxicity in the Dental Office: A Neglected Problem.

D.G. Mantyla, O.D. Wright published *JADA* Vol. 92, June 1976.

Employee exposure criteria, as proposed by NIOSH, are even more stringent than those in UOSHA. The NIOSH document states that "Exposure to inorganic mercury is defined as exposure to a concentration of inorganic mercury greater than 40 percent of the recommended level in the workplace." Therefore, any value exceeding this figure creates an environment of mercurial exposure for those in the workplace.

Medical records of employees must be available for authorized review for at least five years after an employee's last exposure to inorganic mercury.

Comment:
If this NIOSH (National Institute of Occupational Safety and Health) proposal were followed in dentistry, almost every dental office in the country would have to be furnishing records of employees. (Many offices are well above the maximum level as it is.) They are seldom concerned about these high levels much less concerned about being at 40 percent of the maximum.

Experimental Design In the Clinical Evaluation of Amalgam Restorations.

J. Goldberg, et.al. published *J. Biomed Mat. Res.* 14 (6): 777-778 1980.

In evaluations of amalgam restorations, design parameters have included alloy, operator, type of tooth, type of restoration, number of restored surfaces, size of the restoration, patient effects, condensation technique, compressive strength, microhardness, anodic polarization, tensile strength and static creep.

Comment:
Do you feel an imbalance toward the mechanical aspects of the filling and a partial vacuum where patients (the recipients) are concerned?

The Mercury Enigma in Dentistry.

Wilmer B. Eames published *JADA* Vol. 92., June 1976.

The patient should avoid contact with the mercury compound, be given nutritional guidance, and be prescribed a drug regimen that will enhance the urinary excretion of mercury.

Comment:
At the time this was written (1976), Dr. Eames was listing the "maximum allowable limit of mercury in urine as 150 micrograms per liter. Standards set by the Centers for Disease Control are 30 micrograms. Dr. Eames published in 1983 that up to 500 micrograms was safe. CDC comment on the new level was, "It looks like an accommodation for sloppy procedures."

Eames differs from other authors and the ADA council in fearlessness toward scrap amalgam. He reports:

When disturbed, the scrap elicits high meter readings for mercury vapor concentrations but this high level remains for only a few moments. The surfaces of mercury droplets are covered with particles of dust and silver alloy, and the container should not need to be covered or kept in a refrigerator, nor do its contents need to be covered with water.

Also contrary to ADA recommendations, Eames states:

Although carpeting in the operatory does not prevent high levels of mercury vapor, it does not necessarily contribute to them either.

Comment:
The thing many dentists, including myself, find hard to believe in light of

cautions of higher temperature producing greater vapor is Eames statement on amalgam removal:

The high speed removal of old amalgam restorations without water spray: We believe this to be an insignificant source of contamination.

Comment:
University scientists who publish research data are generally expected to write about specific proofs, not beliefs.

Mercury Intoxication In a Dental Surgery Following Unreported Spillage.

D.P. Mayfield, et.al. published *Brit. Dent J.* 141: 179-186, Sept. 21, 1976.

From the cases reported here, it appears that rapid intake of mercury results in the clinical symptoms of headache, nausea, and diarrhea even with relatively low urine mercury levels. Recovery is prolonged even after short exposure, and in these four cases, significant amounts of mercury were still being excreted eight months after exposure. The first dentist still had abnormally high blood pressure 15 months after the onset of symptoms; it is probable that an underlying essential hypertension was aggravated by the mercury intoxication.

Mercury Poisoning in Dental Practice

I.I. Ship, I.M. Shapiro published Release from School of Dental Medicine, Univ of Penn. March 1983.

Comment:
In this study 298 dentists, age 50 and over, were divided into two groups. One group, the control group, had low levels of mercury as detected by X-ray fluorescence of the head and wrist. The other group showed higher levels of mercury. Neither group had ever complained of any signs or symptoms of heavy metal toxicity.

The article:
The group of dentists with the lowest levels of mercury (control group) showed no evidence of neurological deficits. Of great interest was the finding that the average sural nerve sensory and the average median nerve motor conduction velocities in the experimental group were significantly slower than in the controls (probability level was less than 0.05). In addition, the high mercury experimental group had significantly longer laten-

cies than the control group, especially in the motor component of the median nerve. When values obtained for the individual dentists were compared with those of laboratory controls, further abnormalities were noted. Thus, there was evidence of the Carpal Tunnel Syndrome in five dentists in the group with elevated mercury levels. There was no evidence of this syndrome in dentists in the low mercury control group.

Polyneuropathies, defined as reduced motor or sensory conduction velocities, or response amplitudes in more than two nerves were found in seven dentists. These dentists were also in the elevated mercury group.

All dentists participating in this study had high I.Q.'s. However, when the high and low mercury groups were compared, there were no differences in mean I.Q.'s. The Bender-Gestalt and other neuropsychological tests, revealed statistically significant differences in neuropsychological performance. These were characterized by deterioration in the visual graphic performance of dentists with elevated mercury levels. Furthermore, in the test of perceived health symptoms a higher frequency of dentists with elevated mercury levels scored in the abnormal range. Difference between groups was statistically significant using the Chi-square test. This finding indicated that the mercury exposed group of dentists expressed higher levels of health anxiety than did the controls.

The results of the study indicate that the current standards of mercury hygiene in dentistry are not consistent with safety in the dental office. It is also likely that available knowledge concerning mercury hygiene is not being effectively disseminated or applied.

In addition to the neurological deficits, there was evidence of mild neuropsychological impairment in the high mercury containing group. Thus, mercury absorption was associated with problems in both the central and the peripheral nervous systems. Together, these effects indicate that exposure to mercury over long intervals of time is a serious problem in dental offices, and that a substantial number of practicing dentists and their auxiliary personnel are at risk.

Dentists should re-examine the architecture and decor of their offices, and implement changes to eliminate the most obvious sources of contamination. Much of this can be achieved through the elimination of carpeting, and replacing it with non-porous, unseamed materials. In a related study, carpeting was found in 50 percent of dental offices visited, and represented a major reservoir of mercury.

**(1) Electromotive Forces and Electric Currents Caused by
Metallic Dental Fillings.**

W. Schriever, L.E. Diamond published *J. Dent Res.* 1952, 31, 205-229.

(2) The Mechanism of Marginal Fracture of Amalgam Fillings.

K.D. Jorgensen published *Acta. Odont. Scand.* 1965, 23, 347-389.

(3) Corrosion of Gold and Amalgam Placed in Contact With Each Other.

T. Fusayama, et.al. published *J. Dent. Res.* 1963, 42, 1183-1197.

(4) *Physical Chemistry,* Editor, Moore, W.J., 4th Ed., Longmans, Lond.
1966.

In contact with gold, the rate of corrosion is considerably increased.
Since 1941 the use of amalgam and gold in contact has been warned
against, and since 1952 for serious pathological conditions in the mouth
and hypersensitivity reactions caused by released metallic ions.

"Because of its almost universal toxic effects and the slow onset of symptoms, mercury can probably be considered one of the worst poisons im-
aginable. In 2 grams of amalgam there is more than 30,000 TIMES the
maximum permissible daily intake of mercury (Swedish values)." Dr.
Mats Hanson — Univ of Lund, Sweden.

Comment:
*The statements made above are found in numerous articles and books
throughout the literature. We have chosen just a few of them to be listed
here.*

*As concerns the last statement made, many individual fillings weigh two
grams or more.*

**Systemic Mercury Levels Caused by Inhaling Mist During High-speed
Amalgam Grinding.**

D.E. Cutright, et.al. published *J. Oral Med.* Vol. 28, No. 4, Oct.-Dec. 1973

A total of 48 animals were exposed as described above to the amalgam
mist. Six were used as controls, 6 were sacrificed at 0 hours, 8 hours, 16,
24, 32, 48, and 72 hours post exposure. At the time of sacrifice the brain,

kidneys, heart, lungs, liver and a sample of blood were collected for analysis.

The lungs of the control rats contained an average of 112.3 nanograms of mercury per gram of tissue. This compares to an average of 5060.7 for 0 hours (immediately after exposure), 2753.3 average for 8 hours, 1444.3 for 32 hours, 731.5 for 24 hours, 503.5 for 32 hours, 406.3 for 48 hours and 316.2 for 72 hours.

Analysis of the heart samples revealed an average for the control of 50.72. This rose very rapidly to an average of 4113.1 for the 0 hours. The average fell to 2301.6 at 8 hours, 929.6 at 16 hours and continued to fall to 293.4 at 72 hours.

The average of the control brains was 98.12. This compared to 428 for the 0 hour samples, 460 at 8 hours, 711 at 16 hours, the highest level, and decreased to 266.5 at 72 hours.

Comment:
Picking again on Dr. Eames, consideration of amalgam dust as "insignificant", we think this study raises questions to challenge that.

We find it interesting that physically, seriously ill patients feel markedly better as each filling is removed, even at a single appointment. Evidence presented here certainly shows greater exposure in vital organs.

Perhaps the change in electrical pattern by removing negative electrical current fillings has more benefit than we can measure. Electricity may be the big part of metal toxicity.

Certainly the doctor and assistant should be aware that their hearts, lungs, and brains can potentially be exposed many times each day. Here we have more compassion for the doctor and assistant than the patient. The patient can go home. (Of course, he takes his fillings with him.)

Chronic Effects of Mercury on Organisms

I.M. Trachktenberg, National Institutes of Health, DHEW Publication No. (NIH) 74-473, 1973.

The author in his review and in the series of his own clinical observations of industrial workers exposed to low levels of mercury associates symptoms of fatigue, headache, vegetative neurosis, motor weakness, hypotension and cardiorespiratory distress with "micromercurialism". He develops the hypothesis that in micromercurialism there is "a series of latent changes, especially biochemical, neurohumoral, and immunobiological in nature..." which "do not cause gross somatic disturbances, rather they are reflected in delicate reflex and metabolic shifts." He notes that there is no correlation of these findings and urinary excretion of mercury.

A. Stock assumed that the development of mercury poisoning is diagnosed less often than had previously been thought. Thus, he postulated, as did Pascal and Faraday, who used mercury in their laboratories, that exposure through time led to heavy mercury intoxication. It is known that Faraday used mercury as a cathode in electrolysis. He developed psychic disturbances, acute asthenia and loss of memory. Despite treatment in a psychiatric hospital, he was practically incapable of developing and participating in scientific activity.

Mercury is easily disseminated in the air of buildings and afterwards is found not only near its place of constant use, but quite far removed from it. Mercury vapor penetrates the pores of the body comparatively easily, and this property of mercury vapor called itself to the attention of hygienists as often "... there appear to be cases of poisoning through the walls" (B.B. Koyranskiy, 1923).

From this, attention is called to the fact that at temperatures of 30-40 degrees C. at the surface of mercury a concentration of its vapors exceed the maximum permissible quantity for industrial sites 3,000-6,000 times, and at temperatures of 60-80 degrees C. the temperature of tool surfaces in shops using mercury, by thirty thousand-eighty thousand times.

Changes in viscosity and absorption spectra of high polymer DNA solutions depend on the presence of certain metal ions, in this case, mercury. It is known that DNA molecules in reactions with $HgCl_2$ decrease significantly and, under the effect of bound mercury reagents, increase (S. Katz, 1958). Accordingly one can say that complexed metal ions, particularly mercury, in reactions with nucleic acids produce reversible changes in the physical properties of the latter and that study of these reversible reactions "can have great significance in explaining the biological function of nucleic acids" (M. Ya. Shkol'nik, 1963) and can additionally elucidate the role of metals as bioelements.

There is another point of view which explains the absorption of mercury in the lungs by stating that mercury vapor dissolves in fluid on the surface of the lungs and from there enters the blood as protein compounds — mercury albuminates. In this, corresponding law of solubility of gaseous substances in liquids determines the rate and quantity of mercury entering the blood; this depends on its relative concentration in air and blood.

Absorbed mercury, entering the stomach, causes the solution of mercury compounds in sodium chloride facilitating their transformation into complex compounds, chloroalbuminates. The latter are large complex molecules, in which mercury preserves its ionized state and carries a positive electrical charge.

Simultaneously metallic mercury, having entered the blood, remains "toxically indifferent". The explanation of this is that particles of mercury, circulating in the blood, though not small, are nevertheless larger than the protein molecules. Upon entering the blood, they are covered by a protein film, which adsorbs on them, taking the role of a protective colloid. Apparently, this factor is responsible for the low toxicity of metallic mercury circulating in the blood.

After analyzing the preceding data and comparing it with the results of his own observations, L.I. Medved' (1946) pointed out the difference in the action mechanism of inorganic mercury salts and their organic derivatives. Inorganic salts in the first moment of entry into the body form chloroalbuminates and are not absorbed by the cells, acting on the excretory tract. Simultaneously, the organic compounds are absorbed and retained in the tissues producing their toxic effect. Evidently, later, under the effects of various complex factors, organic compounds react with the body, change to chloroalbuminates, and after separating from them, exert the same effects as the inorganic salts. Consequently, the processes of mercury transformation in the organism depends upon the route and character of its entry. Organic mercury compounds and their vapors have toxicological features determined by the physical and chemical properties of mercury and its derivatives and by their chemical changes in the body. Therefore, remember that one mechanism underlies all traits and differences in the effects of mercury and its inorganic and organic derivatives, the presence in them of a thiol nucleus, the inactivation of functional groups (especially sulfhydryl) of cellular proteins.

Special note should be made of the fact that mercury can leave its depot and enter the blood over a prolonged period many years after cessation of all contact with it. It can cause depression in the general functional state of the body under the effect of harmful factors.

Cases of mercury poisoning in the newborn are known if the nurslings ingest mercury compounds. The literature described such a case in which completely healthy persons drank milk from cows which had been rubbed with a mercury ointment. The people showed signs of intoxication (stomatitis, stomach pains, diarrhea).

V.N. Chernigovskiy (1949) found that chemoreceptors are related to tissue receptors. In other words, they "intercept" shifts not only in blood chemistry, but in tissue metabolism of substances. This is why changes in tissue trophics develop frequently as a consequence of enzyme reactions affected by thiol poisons, including mercury, which are complex irritants of chemoreceptors. Additionally, toxic substances blocking thiol enzyme systems, alter the metabolism of the nerve endings themselves (Kh. S. Koshtoyants, 1945, S.V. Anichkov, 1953, M.L. Belen'kiy, 1951, V.N. Chernigovskiy, 1949).

Electrocardiographic studies made at the beginning of exposure, and then after 16-95 days (first series) and 90-329 days (second series). In the latter case electrocardiograms (EKG) were taken during the simultaneous modeling of coronary insufficiency and measured three standard responses. The results were compared with initial quantities and also with analogous electrocardiographic data taken from healthy rabbits (A.O. Saytanov, 1960). First of all we noted the absence of any EKG indicator changes before the beginning of the experiment (basic data). In all cases experimental rabbits had normal EKG's with a predominance of the right hand type of distribution of the electric axis. During the first 3-4 weeks thereafter the EKG's remained unchanged. Then tachycardia, and diminished cardiac contraction frequency was noted. By the third month all test rabbits had developed pronounced bradycardia in which the heart rate of the majority of animals did not exceed 220-250 beats per minute. Changes were characterized by lowering and broadening of P voltage waves. In the ventricular complex there was a decrease in R and T voltage waves and in some cases, displacement of the ST interval.

The most noticable changes were in beat frequency and voltage. Thus, by the end of the second month the cardiac contraction rhythm reached a maximum — 310/min. By the 70th day it had decreased to 252/min (marked bradycardia). Notable changes occurred in P voltage, from an average of 0.12 mv it had decreased to 0.05 mv by the 70th day. R Voltage showed a definite change from 0.36 mv to 0.24 mv by the end of the experiment. A more significant dimunition occurred in S voltage from an average initial 0.21 mv to 0.09 mv by the end of the experiment. T went from 0.25 mv to 0.17 mv.

Currently, many facts have accumulated indicating that cardiac function usually depends on cholinoreceptor properties. The vagus nerve endings contain acetylcholine having a highly specific effect on the heart muscle which incorporates cholinoreceptors — proteins, the active principle of which are SH- groups. The SH- group reaction capacity is affected by mercury and can change aspects of acetylcholine formation and tissue response to it. That is why we can conclude that the mercury effects produce specific shifts both in the biochemical dynamics of the cardiac muscle and in its response, despite the latter displaying (in origin and course) "non-specific" type reactions.

Changes in heart action under the influence of mercury, evidently, is much connected with mercury's direct action on the heart itself and on its metabolism of substances. In some experiments there was a divergence between the degree of development of the extra-cardiac effect, as, for example, bradycardia and the degree of shift in other EKG components, especially in the final part — of the ST, interval and R and T peaks. Pathomorphological data, to be discussed in the following chapter, confirms this. Changes followed in animals exposed to low mercury concentrations included granular dystrophy of the myocardium, dystrophic changes in the capillary endothelium (desquamation and swelling), disorders in coronary blood formation. Our experiments showed that the heart is a notable mercury depot.

Functional disturbance in the myocardium is a consequence of disruption of extracardiac heart activity regulation as a result of the continuous toxic effect of mercury on the myocardium and heart valves, primarily through SH- group blockage. T.M. Turpayev (1950) proposed that "suppression of the contractile properties of the myocardium through the action of thiol poisons occurring as a consequence of SH- enzyme inactivation is directly linked with the energetic contractile act of the myocardium."

Prolonged exposure to mercury inhibits protein resynthesis, depresses the reactive capacity of protein molecules, inactivates free SH- groups of cell proteins. Naturally, these disruptions of protein metabolism must be reflected in morphological changes. Dystrophic changes in organs and tissues are a consequence of metabolic disturbance.

On the basis of the preceding studies and comparison of our results with literature data, it becomes evident that the dynamics of pathological changes arising during micromercurialism play as crucial a role as CNS and consequent vascular disorders with the appearance of hypoxia, thus the effect of mercury on the cardiovascular system, especially, on vascular permeability applies to all organs and tissues. Apparently, both indicated mechanisms are closely linked and mutually affect one another in the course of forming in the organism, affected by mercury, of corresponding morphological disorders.

All those working with mercury, its compounds or mercury-filled instruments, must wear special, protective clothing (hats, coveralls); work with open mercury should be done inside plastic glove boxes or under the hood; clothing must not touch the mercury. Taking special clothing home is absolutely forbidden. Special protective clothing must be made of dense white material which absorbs mercury poorly. Coveralls must be tightly stitched, have no pockets and must be cleaned at least once a week.

Cleaning proceeds as follows: Contaminated clothing or coveralls are freed of dust, loaded into a washing machine and rinsed for thirty minutes with cold water. The rinsed clothing is washed with washing soda-soap solution (4 l/kg clothing) and washed for thirty minutes at 70-80 degrees C., treated with 1-2 percent HCI. Then it is washed in an alkaline solution for 20 minutes at 70-80 degrees C., which frees the fabric of 96-99 percent of its mercury.

Dr. Olympio Pinto spent several years gathering data for his Master's thesis after receiving his dental degree. Eighteen months into a two-year program for his Masters, the National Institute of Dental Research put a stop to his research. He had to drop the project and finish his Masters in the field of anatomy. There is far more impact in the words published here than one can possibly absorb in one reading. I helped assemble this article from his original work from the 60s and have read it probably 15 times over the past 10 years. It is only now taking on its full meaning. I wanted to select the important issues, but could not decide what to leave out, so we are reprinting the whole article. Dr. Pinto is the true mentor of awareness of mercury toxicity.

Mercury Poisoning in America.

O.F. Pinto, H.A. Huggins, published *J. Intl. Acad. Prev. Med.* Vol. 3. No. 2, Dec, 1976.

A century ago it was already becoming difficult for a single scientist to have a full command of the entire intellectual activity of his day. Since that time, science has become increasingly the business of specialists, and the specialties have tended to grow progressively narrower. A century ago there was a Gauss, a Faraday and a Darwin. Today there are few scholars who can call themselves mathematicians, physicists or biologists without restriction. In the fields of the Dental and Medical sciences, due to the progressive deepening and ramification of knowledge, there are no more Dentists or Physicians, but Surgeons, Orthodontists, Prosthodontists, Pathologists, Hematologists, Gastroenterologists, etc., and the men involved in one discipline regard the next discipline as something belonging to his colleague three doors down the corridor. The so-called General Practitioner is no longer interested in collecting scientific information, since his field is limited to the surface of his science. Many times a patient is wrongly referred to a specialist for treatment, and starts an interminable "pilgrimage," frequently finding the right man when it is already too late. To give an example, we could mention the anemic patient who is referred to the Hematologist who sends him back to the General Practitioner, who in turn consults with the Dietician and frequently after achieving no significant improvement, refers the patient once more to a Gastroenterologist. The latter may achieve an artificial improvement by the administration of iron, vitamin B_{12}, etc., or may again refer the patient to a Gynecologist, Urologist, Pathologist, etc. Only seldom will this patient be sent to a

Dentist and in this case it often happens that the Dentist views his part merely as a matter of restoring the occlusion for a better mastication: some time later this same patient may appear with a leukemia and die in the hands of an Oncologist or Pathologist.

The result of a lack of this correlation or holism in science is similar to what occurred when the Oregon Territory was being invaded simultaneously by the United States settlers, the British, the Mexicans and the Russians: an inextricable tangle of exploration, nomenclature and laws.

The purpose of this paper is to present one of these "blank areas of science," or blindspots, in an attempt to elucidate some aspects of certain diseases of unknown or unclear etiology that might well be related to the field of Dentistry.

Suspected Action of Mercury in Human Metabolism

Amalgam Restorations Are Common

Despite the frequent appearance of citations in the Medical and Dental literature considering the relationship of amalgam to systemic diseases, there is no scientific proof either to affirm or deny this. Considerable literature is available on amalgam research, but these data are related only to its physical properties. No one seems to have studied its compatability with the human organism.

There is no doubt that amalgam is the most widely used restorative material in dentistry. Shoonover and Sounder (1950) state that "more restorations are made from amalgam than from all other materials combined." Roper (1947) mentioned that 68,170,326 permanent fillings were made by U.S. Army dentists from December 7, 1941 to September 1, 1945 and that most of them were amalgam. This considers only the Army dentists in a period of less than four years. What would the total number be for the whole country, still more, the whole world?

Delayed Expansion

Sweeney (1944) states that the "delayed expansion" of amalgam continues indefinitely. Shoonover, et al. (1942) found that amalgams sometimes showed blistering of their surfaces and that this phenomenon was due to the formation of gas within the filling as the result of galvanic corrosion. They proved that galvanic action was responsible for the "delayed expansion," and large quantities of gas were shown to be contained within these amalgams. The gas was shown to be hydrogen and its pressure within the filling was shown to be between 1,600 and 2,200 pounds per square inch.

The existence of galvanic current and electrolysis in the mouth has been discussed for nearly a century (Patrick, 1880). Lain, Schriever and Caughron (1940) wrote that there is almost unanimous agreement that:

1. The human saliva constitutes a good electrolyte.

2. In every oral cavity containing dissimilar metals all the elements of galvanic cells are present, and

3. That certain symptoms and pathologic lesions in the mouth diagnosed as electrogalvanic lesions disappear after complete and correct replacement with certain metals.

Shoonover and Sounder (1941) investigated the rate of corrosion of dental alloys under various conditions and state:

"One has only to examine the surface and base of any dental fillings to observe corrosion, which is probably the result of galvanic action. Such amalgams need not be in contact with another metal or in mouths containing additional metal fillings. . ."

and further:

"Galvanic action on a single metal filling may also result from exposure of different areas of the filling to solutions that are not chemically the same. Such a condition produces a simple concentration cell, which in dental practice would be found where an amalgam would be exposed to a solution of a different concentration, for example of oxygen, from that in contact with the surface."

Schriever and Diamond (1952) described another way in which a single filling within the mouth may act to produce a galvanic current and consequently corrosion. They describe the filling as a single metal between two electrolytes in contact externally with the saliva and internally with the fluids of the tooth, bone and tissues which they call the "bone fluid." Since these two electrolytes are in turn in contact with each other through the tissues, a "liquid junction cell" is established, and an electric current exists in that circuit.

There are other ways also in which a single amalgam filling may produce galvanic cells. Strader (1949), Lane (1949) and Harper (1928) state that different parts of the same filling are different "metals." The amalgam filling is a complicated crystalline mass made up of different combinations and forms of the metals comprising it. This complex mixture is bathed by saliva, which is an electrolyte. Different areas of the same filling may act as anode and cathode and the saliva as electrolyte.

Mumford (1957), in his research, found that:

1. Different dental fillings (metal) immersed in saliva, serum and in whole blood generated similar values in millivolts (from 0 to 639), and were similar in each of the three electrolytes.

2. Changing the distance, area of cross section, and the area of the electrodes in contact with the electrolyte, left the E.M.F. approximately constant.

3. Raising the temperature in the cell increased the E.M.F. and the increase was similar for saliva and serum.

4. When the current was measured by a microammeter, the cell polarized rapidly. The cell recovered when the circuit was interrupted, but not completely.

Amalgam and Clinical Symptoms

Meyer (1938) mentioned a case of significance in which:

"The patient complained of burning sensations in the tongue, digestive upsets, dryness of the mouth and throat, inflammation of the gums, poor appetite, weakness and numbness of the hands and feet, general discomfort, lack of interest, depression, disturbed sleep and loss of weight.

"The disproportion of slightly abnormal physical findings and the patient's numerous complaints were striking. The blood picture was atypical, with a high leukocyte count and a low percentage of hemoglobin.

"In the search for the cause of symptoms, several old copper amalgam fillings were discovered and removed. Examination of the urine just prior to the extraction of the teeth showed 0.004 mg of mercury in a 24-hour specimen of 1.5 liters.

"Within a few weeks after removal of teeth, all symptoms had disappeared, with the exception of slight burning sensations of the mouth and tongue, and the patient was restored to good health."

Many other cases were mentioned, similar to these; cases of dermatitis, sore throat, swelling joints, fever, malaise, albumin and casts in the urine, in which the patient's condition varied from better to worse for about six months, until the amalgam fillings were removed. Metallic ions from metal fillings were found included in oral tissues.

Considering that the finished amalgam restoration contains an average of 45 percent to 50 percent mercury, we can understand how chronic poisoning may occur as corrosion takes place. We know that mercury bichloride can cause ulcerations in the mucosa of the stomach if ingested, even in small amounts. Why should not a gastric ulcer result from the combination of mercury from dental fillings with gastric juice and its hydrochloric acid? Which organs would be affected and what signs and symptoms would appear?

Bichloride of mercury has effects which depend on the dosage and the length of time. In some cases, there may be corrosion of the stomach and duodenum, severe destruction of renal tubular epithelium may also occur with calcium deposition in the necrotic tubules.

In pernicious anemia (the cause of which is not fully understood), Castle (1955) suggested that the substance present in the normal gastric juice (intrinsic factor) in combination with certain protein substances (extrinsic factor) produces a material which he has called the "hematopoietic principle" or "erythrocyte maturing factor" and which is necessary for normal red cell production.

In the patient suffering from pernicious anemia the intrinsic factor is absent. Would mercury be interfering with this?

Hyams and Harry (1933) state:

"Human saliva, whether acid, alkaline or neutral makes a good electroyte through which metallic electrons freely circulate from a metal of higher to one of lower electropotential."

Solomon, Reinhard and Goodale (1933) have shown, however, that there is no direct connection between the amount of current measured and the clinical symptoms present.

Enzymatic Activity and Heavy Metals

From the available literature, it seems that attempts have been made to relate not only failure in the use of certain restorative materials, but also some important systemic diseases to galvanism in the oral cavity. However, it is of crucial significance to consider the importance of the heavy metals in the gastrointestinal tract as enzyme inhibitors, since enzymes are of fundamental importance in proper digestion so vital to the maintenance of physiological, organic balance.

White and co-authors (1959) state in their textbook of biochemistry:

"The significance of gastric urease in relation to ammonia formation from urea and the part these play in neutralizing gastric juice in normal human beings and in certain cases of peptic ulcer have been studied in some detail (Fitzgerald, O. and Murphy, P., *Irish J. Med. Sci.*, 6th Series, 97-1950)."

Many of the instances of noncompetitive inhibition are actually examples of combination of inhibitor and enzyme to form chemical derivates in which the combination is essentially irreversible. Sulfhydryl groups are present in some enzymes, and these groups are, in many instances, essential to the enzymatic activity. Heavy metals which form insoluble sulfides also react with sulfhydryl groups to form mercaptides.

Various organic mercury derivates such as p-chloromercuribenzoate and certain arsenicals react with the SH group. Those enzymes which contain essential metal ions are specifically inhibited by compounds which form complexes with the metal.

West and Todd (1957) state:

"The toxicity of mercuric ions is largely due to their combination with the sulfhydryl group (SH) of enzymes with resulting inactivation. Thus it is seen that the physician is constantly confronted with abnormal states which are the result of, or attended by, changes in the chemical reactions within tissues."

According to the same authors:

"Certain heavy metals are classed as enzyme poisons, although they would better be classed as inactivators or inhibitors, since many of the reactions are reversible! Mercury, Silver and Gold are examples."

Absence of free hydrochloric acid in the stomach is a constant finding in anemias, chronic gastritis, carcinoma of the stomach and other diseases occurring with advancing age. Less than one-third of the patients with pernicious anemia die from lesions directly associated with it. Prominent causes of death include complications referrable to the spinal cord, heart disease, cancer, apoplexy, pneumonia, trauma or nephritis. However, simple chronic anemia commonly occurs when associated with chronic infections, heavy metal intoxications, chronic gastrointestinal renal or hepatic diseases and poor hygienic surroundings. In order to be brief, let us say that the signs and symptoms of the diseases of the blood and blood forming organs have *surprisingly curious similarities with those of heavy metal poisoning.*

176

Anderson (1957) states:

"Corrosive sublimate (mercury bichloride) has effects which depend on dosage and length of survival time. In acute cases there is corrosion of the stomach and duodenum, the mucosa of which appears white and opaque. In the colon there is an intensive hemorrhagic and membranous inflammation. If there is survival for a few days or weeks, severe destruction of renal tubular epithelium occurs with calcium deposition in the necrotic tubules. In such cases death usually results from anuria. Schenben and Hausmann have pointed out that mercury poisoning may result in a primary severe vascular injury in limited portions of the intestinal tract."

It seems that in chronic poisoning, all the heavy metals have a similar behavior and follow a similar course in the organism, producing signs and symptoms that are probably common to its group, as intestinal colic, weakness of extensor muscles, anemia, blue line in the gums, mental disturbances, diarrhea, intestinal hemorrhages, etc. It seems also that the heavy metals affect mainly the reticulo-endothelial system and the organs responsible for excretion.

In lead poisoning, the brain, liver, kidneys, bone marrow and spleen are affected. Parathyroid hormone will mobilize the lead from the bones. The same will probably be true for other heavy metals as mercury, tin and silver.

Traces of silver, as mentioned before, would inhibit urease probably interfering with the breakdown of urea in ammonia and carbon dioxide. As a consequence the urea level would be raised in the blood.

Poisoning by heavy metals, such as mercury bichloride and other corrosives, may produce an intense hemorrhagic and diphtheritic inflammation of the bowel. The ileum and colon are most markedly involved. In uremia no particular substance or toxin is known to be the cause.

If the phosphorus level in the blood is raised, there will be a parallel hyperactivation of the parathyroid glands, with consequent osteoporosis which, as mentioned before, could be related to Hodgkin's disease, leukemias, pernicious anemia, etc.

Dental Fillings and Heavy Metal Poisoning?

In confronting such symptoms, what physician or even specialist would normally think in terms of chronic heavy metal poisoning from dental fillings? What "General Practitioner" of medicine normally knows enough of the dental science to raise such suspicion? What Dermatologist would normally seek the root of a skin allergy in dental fillings? Who would ask for a blood, urine or stool analysis with the specific purpose of detecting heavy metals? Even the dentists themselves do not realize this, since generation after generation they have been taught that the amalgam is an excellent restorative material, because (Simon, 1956) amalgam has been shown by experience and research to be completely non-irritating to pulpal tissue — the conservative cavity if used for the amalgam restoration minimizes the response to heat and cold, and amalgam restorations are made in one continuous operation which subjects the tooth's vital structure to minimal injury. Besides that, its cost is one of the most important factors for the wide use it has today.

Of course the fact that the most important diseases have been diagnosed after the appearance of the amalgam in dentistry is in part due to the fact that we are becoming better diagnosticians and better diagnostic weapons become more available every day. However, we should also regard very carefully any vestige of evidence left whenever we talk in terms of research, particularly when it is related to human health.

According to Goldberg (see reference), amalgam was first introduced in the United States in 1825. McGehee (1956) and co-authors state that the first silver amalgam is supposed to have been introduced by Bell of England in 1819 and later used by Traveau in Paris in 1826.

In a review of the history of medicine it is recorded that nephritis was first recognized in 1827, Hodgkin's disease in 1832, leukemia in 1845, Addison's disease in 1849, Banti's disease in 1881, Gaucher's disease in 1882, anorexia nervosa in 1888, Dercum's disease in 1892, Van Jaksch's anemia in 1890, sickle cell anemia in 1910, chronic monocytic leukemia in 1913, to mention only a few.

Another curious fact is that the above-mentioned diseases are all of unclear or unknown etiology, presenting at the same time many common symptoms with chronic heavy metal poisoning, as it is the case of a diffuse and irregular osteoporosis of the calvarium that appear in Hodgkin's disease, sickle cell anemia, leukemia and blood dyscrasias of the childhood.

If all the heavy metals follow a similar course in the organism, the *products of corrosion of dental alloys* would probably be deposited in the bone marrow, liver, spleen, etc., causing a stimulation or irritation (who knows?) in the bone marrow that would correspond to hypertrophic changes, parallel to the enzyme inhibition in the gastrointestinal tract that might progress toward an uremia, hyperparathyroidism, etc., by interference with the water and electrolyte balance, renal tubules, etc., as mentioned before. As it occurs in lead poisoning the parathyroid glands would be hyperactivated in an organic attempt to remove the foreign substance from the bone marrow.

As Comroe (see reference) and co-authors pointed out:

". . . The animal body should be regarded as a highly organized, highly specialized, delicately balanced and subtilely motivated biochemical plant, made up of departments intimately connected, correlated and coordinated."

Thus, any aggression to the gastrointestinal tract will cause deep changes in all others; and while it is not the purpose of the present paper to consider the corrosion of dental alloys as the root of all the diseases mentioned herein, it is our purpose to raise a hypothesis worthy of research and review.

Collins (1959) in a very recent article presented a very exciting hypothesis on the etiology of leukemia and he states:

"Clinical observation of acute leukemia of lymphatic type following immunological procedures started a train of thought which led to the hypothesis that leukemia is an abnormal or pathologically excessive response to an antigen or prolonged antigenic stimulation which may be electively administered or may result from environmental hazards.

"I suggest the following sequence of events in the genesis of leukemia: In response to an antigen, antibody is formed. This can go on until maximal antibody production has been reached. Thereafter, continued presence of the antigen leads eventually to hyperplasia of antibody producing cells and consequent exhaustion with the production of abnormal cells, the abnormality being a depletion of some 'identity protein,' loss of which confers on the cell the property of unrestricted growth.

"Historically, clinicians have noted the clinical and hematological similarity between acute leukemia and fulminating infections. It has been shown that one of the functions of the spleen is fixation and storage of antigen where it gives rise to prolonged stimulant effect. The difference between stimulation and irritation is merely one of degree."

Due to the fact that in this type of chronic poisoning the metals are probably interfering with the elaboration of vital substances in the gastrointestinal tract, and are being spread throughout the organism by the circulatory system, toxic effects may be evident everywhere in the organism. These effects may be due either to a deviation in the biochemical reactions indispensable to the body economy, or due to local stimulation or irritation at the site of absorption, excretion or deposition: it is unfortunate that clinical analyses are seldom made to detect these metals in the excretions, and that they are very rarely diagnosed as a causative factor of any known disease of unknown etiology. Besides that, the amount of metallic ions usually shown in these tests is so minute that it is generally discarded or neglected as an etiologic factor; however, it seems that in cases of chronic poisoning, the clinical analyses are often of questionable value since the organism can retain some poisons as by means of its "self-detoxifying" organs. Obscure symptoms of weakness, anorexia, skin changes, pallor, diarrhea, dizziness, thirst, edema, etc., could either indicate intoxication or infection: in fact, in the same way that acute poisoning many times imitates acute infections in several aspects, chronic poisoning may also imitate chronic infections or diseases in most of their clinical aspects, because essentially the aggression is chemical. On the other hand, there is also the possibility that part of these metals may combine with calcium salts and deposit in the bones, failing to show in the clinical analysis. Temporary improvement may be attained by the specialist by detecting and compensating for the resultant metabolic deficiency in the organs that are related to his field; but, as the source is not removed, the condition acquires a cyclic character, with reincidence shortly after interruption in the medication. It seems that this mechanism follows a progressive course (either due to cumulative effects or to selective, mild and constant stimulation and irritation in the same organs), until it reaches the point that it causes an atrophy or hypertrophy of the tissues involved, establishing then a definite pattern of the disease. In this regard, Collins (1959) mentioned in his article:

"Attempts to transmit leukemia from man to man, even by blood transfusion , have not been successful. This is not surprising if the concept that leukemia is an abnormal response to antigenic stimulation is correct."

Moreover, Menkin (1957) has shown that substances present in inflammatory exudate are capable of causing either hyperplasia or hypoplasia of the myeloid marrow; that the mechanism governing the release of excess cells in hyperplasia appears to depend on the presence of an intact spleed, and that maximal antibody production may well hamper this mechanism. Inflammation would be the first organic response to a strange substance depositing in the bones. This, however, is a subject that must be established by an extensive research, since no literature could be found detailed enough to contain a complete dental record of the patient with systematic diseases suspected to be related to chronic heavy metal poisoning.

Yet another fact of relative importance to the understanding of the present hypothesis is that the salivary glands seem to play an important role in excreting mercury (and other metals also) in systemic poisoning. If this is true, it would explain, in part, the mechanism of cumulative effects, as well as the cyclic character of certain diseases of chronic aspect with intercurrent symptoms of acute form. Here the observation becomes questionable, since the patients could not be left without any medication, in which case the symptoms of a probable poisoning effect were modified, or even disappeared temporarily. And, too, another fact that is constantly challenging the observer's curiosity is that B.A.L. (British anti-lewisite: 2, 3, mercaptopropanol) is well known for its anti-toxic properties and is widely used in cases of arsenic and heavy metal poisoning. Finally, another compound of the mercaptans group (6, mercaptopurine. Purinethol, an analogue of hypoxantine and of adenine) is employed in the treatment of acute leukemia in children. The presence of a thiol group, -SH, in the compounds of the mercaptans group seems to be responsible for its anti-toxic effects, since it is possible that here again the -SH radical is displaced by the heavy metals, in the same way that happens with the group of enzymes containing an -SH radical. In that way, B.A.L. would act as a carrier in the excretion of the poisonous substance.

As such heavy metal poisoning progresses without removal of this source of enzymic inhibition (stimulant or irritant), slow-developing but constantly increasing changes seem to appear in the organism, either as a result of a nutritional deficiency (i.e., atrophic changes in the oral mucosa, angular cheilosis, atrophy of the papillae of the tongue, etc.), or due to local irritation (i.e., hypertrophic gingivitis, periodontosis, atrophy of the gastric mucosa, tumor of the gastric mucosa, atrophy or tumor of the intestinal mucosa).

Here it is interesting to note that the more the patient's condition aggravates, the closer contact he maintains with the "specialist" and the more distant he is from the dentist (either by financial problems or by the presence of health problems of more urgent nature). At the time that the patient is referred to the dentist, most often for complete removal of the teeth, it is already too late, since the patient's organism has undergone irreversible pathological changes (i.e., arteriosclerosis, hepatic cirrhosis, atrophy of the gastric mucosa, chronic glomerulo-nephritis, etc.).

Cellular Dysfunction

Again, returning to the enzymatic inhibition in the gastrointestinal tract, as mentioned before, the heavy metals have an inhibitory effect upon enzymes of the sulfhydryl group, and this may lead to an interference with the mechanism of oxidation and reduction within the organism's cells. The Krebs cycle is perhaps one of the most important chemical phenomena that occur within the living organism; co-enzyme A that is posteriorly changed to acetyl-co-enzyme A is one of the compounds that contains the sulfhydryl (-SH) radical, which is inhibited in the presence of heavy metals such as Hg and Ag. If co-enzyme A is inhibited, the cholesterol formation is disturbed, which is important in the production of vitamin D, bile salts and steroid hormones. Vitamin D is well known for its importance in the mechanism of retention or deposition of calcium and phosphorus salts in the bones. Sodeman (see reference) states that:

> "It is synthesized in the body through irradiation of skin, and in the adult in normal circumstances an unknown and probably chief source is endogenous."

Moreover, since cholesterol is a precursor of vitamin D, any disturbance in its metabolism would probably interfere with the biosynthesis of vitamin D. Bile salts are also known to be indispensable in the absorption of fat-soluble vitamins (A, D, E, K). Steroid hormones are also of crucial importance in the total organic balance. Finally, another possible site of interference exerted by the heavy metals within the citric acid cycle would be in the succinyl co-enzyme A, which is essential in the synthesis of the porphyrins, hence of hemoglobin.

The possibility that heavy metals corroded from dental alloys may be interfering with vital metabolic reactions within the human body, and the mechanisms of action of these "anti-metabolites" are of such complexity and extension, that special research would be indispensable for the evaluation of this hypothesis, as well as to investigate its veracity.

Conclusion

When science arrives at the cutting edge between living organisms and chemicals, there is a strong divergence among scientists of the various fields (i.e., Micro-biologists and Biochemists); and our knowledge often becomes obscure and hypothetical, while diseases become fatal, often with a clinical aspect that many times imitates the organic response to bacterial infection, to viral infection, to allergy, or to poisoning (that is essentially a protein coagulation, or antimetabolic action). It seems that the more science advances in the search for the etiology of cancer, the closer the scientists come to the limit between a biological concept (virus?) and a chemical concept (hormones?), and perhaps nutrition, enzymes, co-enzymes, vitamins and other as important factors will be seen as the next investigatory steps to elucidating the etiology of many obscure diseases. Finally, it is our hope that the hypothesis we have advanced here will be given a full and complete evaluation in our movement towards this more holistic health care orientation.

References[1]

Anderson, W.A.D., *Synopsis of Pathology*, the C.V. Mosby Co., (Fourth Ed.), 198, 1957.

Castle, et al., mentioned in Bernier, J.L., *The Management of Oral Disease*, the C.V. Mosby Co., 343, 1955

Collins, N.J., A concept of the etiology of leukemia, *Bulletin of Cancer Progress*, 9:2, 49, March-April 1959.

Comroe, B.I., Collins, L.H. and Crane, M.P., *Internal Medicine in Dental Practice*, Lea & Febiger, (Fourth Ed.), 261.

Goldberg, M.A., *Materials Used in Dentistry and Their Manipulation*, (Fourth Ed.), 81.

Harper, W.E., Amalgam failures. Where is the fault in the alloy or in the operator??, *Dominion D.J.*, 40:153, May 1928.

Hyams, B.L. and Harry, C.B., Dissimilar metals in the mouth as a possible cause of otherwise unexplainable symptoms, *Canadian Med. Assn. J.*, 29:488, 1933.

Lain, E.S., Schriever, W. and Caughron, G.S., Problem of electrogalvanism in the oral cavity caused by dissimilar metals, *JADA*, 27:1765, November 1940.

Lane, J.R., Survey of dental alloys, *JADA*, 39:414, October 1949.

McGehee, W.H.C., True, H.A. and Inskipp, F.L., *A Textbook of Operative Dentistry*, (Fourth Ed.) McGraw-Hill, 330, 1956.

Menkin, V., Growth-promoting factor in exudates, mechanism of repair and pre-neoplastic-like responses, *Cancer Res.*, 17:963-969, 1957.

Meyer, mentioned in Traub and Holmes, *Arch. of Dermat, and Syph.*, 38:349, 1938.

Mumford, J.M., Electrolitic action in the mouth and its relationship to pain, *J. Den. Res.*, August 1957.

Patrick, J.J.R., Oral electricity and the new departure, *D. Cosmos*, 22:543, October 1880.

Roper, L.H., Restorations with amalgam in the army: an evaluation and analysis, *JADA*, 34:443, April 1, 1947.

Schriever, W. and Diamond, L.E., Electromotive forces and electric currents caused by metallic dental fillings, *J.D. Res.*, 31:205, April 1952.

Shoonover, I.C. and Sounder, W., Corrosion of dental alloys, *JADA*, 28:1278, August 1941.

Shoonover, I.C. and Sounder, W., Research on dental materials at the National Bureau of Standards, H.B.S., Circular 497, Washington, D.C., U.S. Government Printing Office, August 15, 1950.

Shoonover, I.C., Sounder, W. and Beall, J.R., Excessive expansion of dental amalgam, *JADA*, 29:1825, October 1942.

Simon, W.J., *Clinical Operative Dentistry*, W.B. Saunders Co., 97, 1956.

Sodeman, W.A., *Pathologic Physiology*, (Second Ed.), W.B. Saunders Co., 50.

Solomon, H.A., Reinhard, M.C. and Goodale, H.I., Precancerous oral lesions from electrical causes, *The Dental Digest*, 39:142, 1933.

Strader, K.H., Amalgam alloy: its heat treatment, flow, mercury content and distribution of dimensional change, *JADA*, 38:602, May 1949.

Sweeney, J.T., Manipulation of amalgam to prevent excess distortion and corrosion, *JADA*, 31:375, March 1944.

West, E.S. and Todd, W.R., *Textbook of Biochemistry*, New York, The Macmillan Co., 853, 1957.

White, A., Handler, P., Smith, E.L. and DeWitt, S., *Principles of Biochemistry*, McGraw-Hill Book Co., Inc. 257, 1959.

Hagar, R.N., Schermerhorn, S., Schroeder, C. and Reger, R.H., Mercury hygiene in the dental office, *J. Colo. Dent. Assoc.*, 54:1, 29-36, September 1975.

Hammond, A.L., Mercury in the environment: natural and human factors, *Science*, 171: 3973, 788-789, 1971.

Hepburn, W.B., Behaviour of metal dental fillings in the mouth, *Brit. Den. Journal*, 33: 1131, 1912.

Hernberg, S. and Hasanen, E., Relation of inorganic mercury in blood and urine, *Work, Environment, Health*, 8:ISS 2, 39-41, 1971.

Hollander, L., Galvanic burns of oral mucosa, *JAMA*, 99:383, July 30, 1932.

Hollander, L., Permar, H.H. and Shonfield, L., Leukoplakia of oral mucosa, *JADA*, 20:41, January 1933.

Hyams, B.L., The electrogalvanic compatability of orthodontic materials, *Internat. J. of Orthodont. and Dentistry for Child.*, 19:9, 1933.

Hyams, B.L. and Ballon, H.C., Dissimilar metals in mouths as possible cause of otherwise unexplainable symptoms, *Cana. Maj.*, 28:488, November 1933.

Lain, E.S., Nickel dermatitis, new source, *JAMA*, 96:771, March 7, 1931.

Lain, E.S., Chemical and electrolytic lesion of the mouth caused by artificial dentures, *Arch. Derm. and Syph.*, 25:21, 1932.

Lain, E.S., Electrogalvanic lesions of oral cavity produced by metallic dentures, *JAMA*, 100:717, March 11, 1933.

Lain, E.S. and Caughron, G.S., Electrogalvanic phenomena of oral cavity caused by dissimilar metallic restoration, *JADA*, 23:1641, September 1936.

Lain, E.S., Schriever, W. and Caughron, G.S., Problem of electrogalvanism in the oral cavity caused by dissimilar metals, *JADA*, 1765, November 1940.

Lenhan, J.M., Smith, H. and Harvey, W., Mercury hazards in dental practice, *Brit. Dent. Journal*, 135, 365, 1973.

Leyva, J.C., Alergia del mercurio con dermatitis eczematica causada por calzas de amalgama de plata, Personal Communication, Carrera 10a, 9727, Apt. 302, Bogota, Columbia.

Leyva, J.C., Algunas consideraciones sobre amalgamas dentales, Personal Communication.

Leyva, J.C., A case of hypersensitivity (allergy) for mercury, Personal Communication.

Layva, J.C., Exposicion pro um periodo largo de los dentistas al mercurio, Personal Communication.

Leyva, J.C., Mercurio-quimica y mecanismo de accion, Personal Communication.

Leyva, J.C., Significado para la salud del mercurio usado em pratica dental, Personal Communication.

Lindstedt, G., A rapid method for the determination of mercury in urine, *Analyt.*, 95, March 1970.

Lindstedt, G. and Skare, I., Microdetermination of mercury in biological samples, *Analyt.*, 66:223-229, March 1971.

Lippmann, A., Disorders caused by electric discharges in the mouth with artificial dentures, *Deutsche Med. Wchnschr.*, 56:1394, 1930.

Lu, F.C., Berteau, P.E. and Clegg, D.J., The toxicity of mercury in man and animals, Part of *Tech. Report No. 137*, Mercury contamination in man and his environment, International Atomic Energy Agency, Vienna, Austria (181 p.) 67-86, July 1972.

Manning, P.R., Electrolitic theory of dental caries, *Pac. D. Gaz.*, 26:365, June 1918.

Mantyla, D.G. and Wright, O.D., Mercury toxicity in the dental office: a neglected problem, *JADA*, 92:6, 1189-1194, June 1976.

Mays, C., No battery in a tooth, *Advertizer*, 12:103, 1880.

Morrison, M.A., Electric currents in oral cavity, *Dominion D.J.*, 14:86, January 1902.

184

Mumford, J.M., Electrolitic action in the mouth and its relationship to pain, *J.D. Res.*, 636, 1957.

Nixon, G.S., Mercury in dental surgery, *Br. Dent. Surg. Assist., 29:6, 107-109, 1971.*

Palmer, S.B., *Dental decay and filling materials considered in their electrical relations, Am. J. D. Sc.,* 12:105, 1878.

Palmer, S.B., electrochemical theory, *Am. J. D. Sc.,* 14:166, 1880.

Palmer, S.B., Electricity in the mouth, *D. Items of Int.,* 10:399, September 1888.

Patrick, J.J.R., Oral electricity and new departure, *D. Cosmos,* 22:543, October 1880.

Polia, J.H., What the physicians should know about dental problems, *JADA,* 20:2169, December 1933.

Roome, N.W. and Dahlberg, A.A., Electrochemical ulcer of buccal mucosa (Case Report), *JADA,* 23:1652, September 1936.

Shoonover, I.C. and Sounder, W., Corrosion of dental alloys, *JADA,* 28, August 1941.

Shoonover, I.C. and Sounder, W., Corrosion of Dental Alloys, *JADA,* 28 (Pt. 2), 1278, 1941.

Schriever, W. and Diamond, L.E., Electromotive forces and electric currents caused by metallic dental fillings, *J.D. Res.,* 18:205, 1938.

Schriever, W. and Diamond, L.E., Electromotive forces and electric currents caused by metallic dental fillings, *J.D. Res.,* 31:205, 1952.

Schwisheimer, W., Mercury vapors in dental offices and laboratories: prevention of poisoning, *Zahntchnik,* (Zurich), 29:4, 349-351, 1971.

Smith, Alloys of gallium with powdered metals as possible replacement for dental amalgam, *JADA,* 53:415-424, 1956.

Solomon, H.A. and Reinhard, M.C., Electric phenomena from dental materials, *D. Survey,* 9:23, January 1933.

Solomon, H.A. and Reinhard, M.C., Inhibitory factors in galvanism, *Am. J. Cancer,* 22:606, November 1934.

Solomon, H.A. and Reinhard, M.C., Inhibitory factors in galvanism from dental metals, *D. Cosmos,* 68:1259, December 1936.

Solomon, H.A., Reinhard, M.C. and Goltz, H.L., Salivary influence on galvanism, *D. Items of Int.,* 60;1047, November 1938.

Solomon, H.A., Reinhard, M.C. and Goodale, H.I., Precancerous lesions from electrical causes, *Dental Digest,* 39:149, 1933.

Stallard, H., Silver amalgam as a tooth repair material, Personal Communication, 275, Altamirano Way, San Diego, California.

The treatment of precancerous oral mucous membranes, *Oral Surgery, Oral Med. and Oral Path.,* Col. 13, 1065-1071, 1960.

Ullmann, K., Leukoplakia caused by electrogalvanic current generated in oral cavity, *Ztschr. f. Stomatol.,* 30:802, 868, 1932.

Waerlauz, Z., Tissue reaction to restorative materials, *Oral Surgery, Oral Med. and Oral Path.,* 9:780-791, 1956.

Wakai, E., Potential difference between various kinds of metal applied in oral cavity and their physiologic effects, *JADA,* 23:1000, June 1936.

In this appendix, we are reprinting for you our complete paper as presented to the NIDR/ADA Workshop on Biocompatibility of Dental Materials on July 13, 1984. Immediately following our paper, you will find two separate sets of recommendations as made by the Planning Committee of the Workshop. The first set was given to the journalists at the press conference as a press release immediately following the conclusion of the workshop on Friday, July 13th. The second was sent to us as Workshop participants in August. And finally, we are printing excerpts from the "ADA News", which is a bimonthly newsletter from the American Dental Association.

Systemic Reactions To Silver Amalgam Fillings

Paper Presented to NIDR/ADA Workshop on Biocompatibility of Dental Materials on July 13, 1984 by Hal A. Huggins, DDS.

My first experience speaking to a group such as this was prefaced by a statement made by the moderator. He said, "The world of clinical observation and the world of scientific investigation have always existed on different planets." What I think he was saying is, "East is East and West is West and ne'er the twain shall meet."

Obviously, the people responsible for scheduling this conference do not feel that way. I was asked to present clinical observations relative to the question of mercury toxicity. I would like to extend my gratitude to Dr. Joyce Reese for making this clear to me. She added that it would be the responsibility of the National Institute of Dental Research to determine what methods — if any — need to be employed to confirm or deny the relationship between amalgam and what I have observed in patients.

In reviewing questions I have heard during the past 11 years, I cannot help but relate them to international business trends. One short decade ago America was the leading industrial nation in the world. Today it is taking a back seat to Japan in electronics and in the auto industry.

Business analysts have placed the blame for this loss of supremacy on management attitudes. They say that today's management likes numbers, charts and graphs. They tend to expel the human entity. Japan, they point out, has thrown formulas to the wind and puts emphasis on human interrelationships.

Stewart Emery, author of *Actualizations,* holds a balloon in the aisle that divides his audiences. Half the balloon is painted red and the other half yellow. "What color is this balloon?" he asks as he holds it in the aisle. Half the audience responds "red" and half responds "yellow". His comment is worth remembering: "We often see our differences in reality as a conflict instead of a contribution." (1)

Hayes and Abernathy say, "American managers have increasingly relied on principles which prize analytical detachment and methodological elegance over insight based on experience."(2)

Peters and Waterman in their book *In Search of Excellence* sum up the problem by calling it "Paralysis through Analysis." (2)

I see red-and-yellow-balloon thinking in myself as well as in my colleagues. Last month a group of researchers was in my office. I asked if they wanted to see videotapes of my patients before and after treatment. The answer was an emphatic "No". They were interested in double-blind studies. I asked if double-blind is like shooting at a duck with both eyes closed. None of us was willing to look at the other side of the balloon. I hope that all of us here — clinicians and researchers alike — can set aside our balloons during this conference.

In 1973 I was exposed to the concept of mercury toxicity by Dr. Olympio Pinto of Rio De Janeiro. Back in the 1920s, Dr. Pinto's dentist-father had observed reversal in cases of leukemia, Hodgkin's disease, bowel disorders and a host of other diseases after removing silver-mercury amalgams. He suggested that many of the "incurable diseases" were mimicked diseases and not true diseases at all. A mimicked disease is one that has external manifestations of a true disease but which, in actuality, is a reaction to mercury.

I called the forensic pathologist at St. Francis Hospital, Dr. David Bowerman, and asked for his opinion on what I had heard. His comment was simple and direct. "If dentistry has created a problem, it is the responsibility of dentistry to investigate and correct the problem."

I looked through the dental literature to find opinions on mercury toxicity. I found comments like this 1971 *JADA* editorial: In answer to the question "Are amalgam fillings hazardous to the patient? the answer was given. "The answer is an unqualified NO. Study after study shows the patient undergoes no risk . . . the dentist, yes, but the hazard can be reduced to practically zero."(4)

187

There were no references attached to the "study after study" and I have been unable to find any.

Also in that March 1971 Journal of the ADA I found Chandler's statement: "The amount of mercury vapor emitted from an amalgam is undetectable."(5) Published information like this and many similar statements led me to think that Pinto was wrong. Even as late as 1980 (*JAMA*, Mar 1980), the American Medical Association was saying ". . . the mercury is present in the form of an intermetallic compound and in such a state that it is normally biologically unreactive . . . The ADA Council on Dental Materials requires biological testing of material to determine safety of certified materials."(3)

Dr. Pinto's suggestion to me was to remove the amalgams on anyone with a sustained elevated white blood cell count. Within one month I found a patient with a white cell count that had remained around 11,000 for several years. No cause was identified. This was the figure Pinto had suggested as his maximum acceptable limit. Upon amalgam removal, that level dropped to between 6,000 and 7,000 in subsequent tests over the next few months.

A story of frustration ensued from 1973 to 1979 while an expanding number of suspected mercury toxic patients appeared in my office. Results were sporadic and unpredictable. At best only 10 percent of the patients responded. Disappointments were common, but the successes were highly motivating. Reversal of one case of epilepsy was sufficient to carry us through several months of failures.

Six years later, in 1979, two new avenues of investigation entered our practice and the success ratio took a quantum leap forward. The first of these was the discovery that negative electrical current exists in some amalgam fillings. Electrical current had been identified as early as 1880 by Patrick (6), but to my knowledge no one had divided current into positive and negative charges. The other avenue was a field in which I already had had an exposure — analytical blood chemistry. Not only was the white cell level affected, but all areas of the differential, hemoglobin, red cell count, hematocrit, etc. were affected. Investigations soon expanded to include the following:

Blood profile
CBC with differential

Hair analysis for toxic metals
Urinary mercury excretion
Electrical currents of fillings

Urinary vitamin C excretion
Immune differential with Hoffman optics

Thermography
Fundus photography

Questionnaire for mercury toxic
    symptoms
Complete medical history
Pulse
Temperature
Blood pressure
Patch test for mercury sensitivity

Mercury vapor emission
Urine bacteriological tests
Psychological testing
Whole blood mercury
Electrocardiogram
Electroencephalogram

From observing these areas and correlating changes with patient responses, we have now categorized disease modalities that have responded to amalgam removal from the mouth into five headings. They are as follows:

1. Neurological
2. Cardiovascular
3. Collagen
4. Immunological
5. Allergic

THE POTENTIAL OF MERCURY AS A PROBLEM

Mercury in the mouth has been the subject of controversy for over a century. To establish mercury as a potential problem, it would have to satisfy the following parameters. Mercury would have to:

1. come out of the filling
2. form a compound that is toxic
3. form a sufficient quantity of this material to produce conditions of illness
4. demonstrate remission of the conditions upon amalgam removal

Amalgam is generally composed of mercury, silver, copper, tin and zinc — all metallic compounds with positive valence. In silver-tin amalgam the main phases are Ag_3Sn, Ag_2Hg_3, Sn_8Hg and, after aging $Ag_6Hg_3 \bullet_5 Sn$. In copper-rich amalgams there are Cu_3Sn, Cu_6Sn_5, Cu_3Hg and often an AgCu eutectium.[7] All have the ability to enter into chemical reactions at mouth temperature and all can form one pole of a battery in an electrolyte. Mercury has a high ionization potential (10.39 electron-volts) which explains its tendency to be highly reactive within a conducive electrochemical environment.[8] Saliva forms an excellent electrolyte. There are multiple chemical complexes of these metals when amalgam is formed. All of these compounds are termed "corrosion products" and they can occur in the oral cavity. Specifically, these compounds are Hg_2Cl_2, HgS, $AgCl$, Ag_2S, SnO, $SN(OH)Cl \bullet H_2O$, $CuCl$, Cu_2S and Cu_2O. (9)

Salivary inorganic ions (Cl⁻, SCN⁻, S⁻ and HS⁻) are of special importance because they catalyze both anodic and cathodic electrochemical processes, thus contributing to corrosion reactions.(10)

Especially reactive as a corrosion catalyst is hydrogen sulfide. (11, 12, 13, 14, 15) Black corrosion products often formed on dental amalgams are largely composed of sulfides.(16) Corrosion of amalgam is difficult to study because the oral environment is chemically dynamic. It is in a constant state of flux. In addition, there are many aggravating factors to the process of corrosion that are not readily accessible for *in vitro* studies. Here are some of the more common aggravating factors:

1. High temperature from foods and drinks
   Higher temperatures increase the rate of corrosion which in turn increases the vapor pressure of mercury.

2. Salty and acidic foods
   These can contribute to or accelerate chemical reactions.

3. Rinsing the oral cavity with hydrogen peroxide
   This considerably increases the oxidation rate over simple dissolved oxygen.
   Hydrogen peroxide can even oxidize gold.(17)

4. Voluntary vomiting
   This is a method of weight control practiced for centuries and probably more prevalent than suspected.
   This leaves high HCl, SH and elevated electrical conductivity in the mouth.
   The resultant increased reactions (ten times greater in aerated digestive juice) produce a marked increase in corrosion even though the length of time is relatively short.(18)
   We have noticed extremely detrimental effects of voluntary vomiting on solubility of composites in these patients.

5. Multitudinous bacteria capable of oxidation, reduction and methylation.

The rate of corrosion occurring in fillings can be estimated by measuring the electrical current generated by these fillings in the mouth. Higher electrical currents indicate greater chemical reactivity.

Oral galvanism has been discussed for over a century in dentistry. Patrick described it in 1880.(6) Mumford first published information relating to the size of the restorations. He stated, "Changing the distance, cross section and the area of the electrodes in contact with the electrolyte left the EMF (electromotive force) approximately constant. Raising the temperature increased the EMF."(19)

There are two types of oral galvanism in a mouth containing amalgam. One is the bimetallic cell. The other is from differential aeration cells. In either case, the cathodic process consists of reduction. In bimetallic cells, the anodic process consists of oxidation (corrosion) of the less noble metal. In aeration cells, the anodic process can result in corrosion, but it may also involve oxidation of organic materials in the saliva.(17) Electrochemical conditions are complicated because of the presence of two electrolytes. One electrolyte is saliva and the other is dentinal fluid. Corrosion has been observed both on the amalgam surfaces exposed to the oral cavity and on the amalgam surfaces directly adjacent to the dentin.(20)

Bimetallic cells are those areas of electrical current generated by the reaction between two dissimilar metals. The more noble of the two will become the cathode and the less noble will become the donor anode that dissolves (or corrodes). Of all the metals used in the mouth, gold is the most noble and tin is the least noble. Every amalgam has a large number of bimetallic cells since the various phases of amalgam have different electrical potentials relative to saliva.(17)

Differential aeration cells are areas of current generated because of a differential in oxygen concentration around a single restoration. Areas of high oxygen concentration become the positive (cathode) pole and the negative (anode) pole is formed where the oxygen supply is limited. There are multiple aeration cells on the surface of a single amalgam since oxygen is limited beneath deposits and in the crevices between amalgam and tooth structure.(17)

Differential aeration cells on gold restorations can lead to dissolution of the less noble metals like copper, silver, cadmium and zinc which are added to reduce the alloy's melting point.(21) It is my suggestion that this reaction accounts for the reduction in current that occurs in older cast gold restorations.

Anodic reactions during amalgam corrosion are oxidations of component metals resulting in somewhat soluble oxides, chlorides and sulfides which are continually abraded and reformed.(22) During the anodic formation of SnO and Cu_2O, hydrogen ions are formed on the surface of the amalgam. Most of it is neutralized by cathodically produced hydroxyl ions. Beneath the surface in narrow crevices, however, an enrichment of acid can take place.(7) During crevice corrosion, pH values of 2.0 have been measured. Both hydrogen ions and chloride ions enhance the formation of soluble corrosion products such as $SnCl_2$, $AgCl_2$, $CuCl_2$ and $HgCl_4$, which can be absorbed into the tissue.(17)

As tin, silver and copper selectively dissolve out of amalgam according to their relative nobility, mercury is enriched on the amalgam surface. Evaporation of mercury will increase and the metal (as vapor) can be inhaled. Mercury vapor pressure over newly made amalgam containing 45 percent mercury was 11 percent of the amount of vapor produced by pure mercury. Vapor pressure over fillings with 54 percent mercury was 26 percent that of pure mercury.(26)

A review of the literature provides a diversification of opinion regarding safe encounters with mercury vapor. Switzerland and the USSR accept 0.01 mcg/M^3 as maximum exposure limits. In America, OSHA suggests 0.05 mg/M^3 but requires that medical records be kept and reviewed for five years if vapor levels in work areas exceed 40 percent of that value.(23) Koos and Longo recommend that the exposure level be lowered to 0.01 mg/M^3 for pregnant women. They state that the fetal nervous system rapidly accumulates mercury with embryopathic and neurologic effects occurring at lower levels than those considered toxic for adults.(24)

There is also a wide diversity of information concerning the volatility of mercury vapor from scrap amalgam. Dr. Wilmer Eames, publishing in the June 1976 *JADA,* says that scrap amalgam elicits high vapor meter readings but only for a few seconds. He further states that it soon becomes covered with dust and is then safe. In addition he says that scrap amalgam does *not* require a lid or a water cover.(25) Barkowski opened a scrap amalgam container and measured 110 mcg/M^3.(37) Mayhall states that storage under water virtually eliminates scrap as a source of vapor.(38) Other authors say water provides no deterrent. In our office we tested scrap amalgam averaging one year old with a Bacharach Mercury Sniffer and found 200 mcg/M^3 over the scrap amalgam at room temperature. This same scrap was put in an incubator at 37 degrees C. for one hour and tested again. On the second test, the amalgam was found to emit 540 mcg/M^3 of mercury vapor. Keep in mind that this is more than ten times the maximum allowable limit as set by OSHA. This was without the advantage of an electrolyte. We measured mercury vapor over scrap amalgam covered with water and found vapor levels in excess of OSHA's upper limit. In 1939, Alfred Stock of Germany found levels of over 2 mcg/M^3 in respired air.(27) Gay, et. al., repeated those experiments in 1979 and found 2.8 mcg/M^3. Gay put the situation to task by measuring the vapor after chewing gum. He measured levels as high as 49 mcg/M^3.(28) Our conference colleague, Dr. Carl Svare, in 1981 measured up to 87.5 mcg/M^3 after chewing gum.(29) In our office, vapor has been measured with both the Jerome Gold Film Mercury Analyzer and the Bacharach Mercury Sniffer. We suggest that there are many substances that can increase mercury vapor emission from amalgam. Some of our patients have equaled or exceeded the values reported by Svare.

One point to note in patient observation is the increase of symptoms following food intake. Prime symptoms expressed by mercury toxic patients are headaches and digestive problems. Hanson's comments on axonal transport of mercury vapor from the nasal sinus into the anterior portion of the brain could explain the headaches.(30) Mercury plus the hydrochloric acid in the stomach could contribute to $HgCl_2$ formation. $HgCl_2$ can contribute to gastrointestinal disturbances. Many foods can cause allergic reactions, but allergic reactions do not explain why amalgam removal without major dietary changes can produce marked improvements within less than a week. Considering the vast amounts of aspirin and antacids that are sold in the U.S. today, this area of concern certainly deserves thorough investigation.

It appears that mercury-binding in amalgam should be easy to test. Techniques are available to test amalgams for the percentage of mercury present. Any test result less than 45 percent mercury should be suspect of having lost mercury to the body. Premixed capsules now give us assurance of the same amount of mercury in each mix, but in the past, mercury content was under the doctor's control. Although mercury content can easily vary from 48 to 54 percent, it is assumed that the doctor would want as dry a mix as possible in order to shorten the setting time.

Jaro Pleva, a PhD in corrosion chemistry, analyzed a five-year-old amalgam and found 27 percent mercury present. His methods utilized JEOL scanning electron microscope with EDAX (energy dispersive analysis with x-ray) equipment.(31)

Tests performed in the Department of Toxicology at St. Francis Hospital in Colorado Springs revealed the following information on two fillings of known insertion and removal dates. One was seven years old and the other eleven years old. Both had 36 percent retained mercury when the tests were done in May of 1984. The tests were performed with cold vapor atomic absorption photospectrometry. The filling which was seven years old registered notably higher electrical current than the one which was eleven years old.

Radics (1970) in a report on loss of mercury from amalgams states, ". . . the amount of mercury missing from an outer corroded zone (50-90 micrometers) was calculated to be up to 560 mg in a mouth with many fillings. If the loss had taken place during ten years, the daily dose would have been 150 mcg".(32)

In answer to the question, "Does mercury come out of the amalgam?", it appears that it does.

Composition of the amalgam itself appears to determine the amount of mercury vapor that can be released. Brune, et.al., in 1983 showed that,

"The levels of copper and mercury released from the (high) copper amalgam were approximately *50 times* those of the other amalgam types studied".(48) Copper concentrations studied were 3 percent, 12.6 percent and 31.3 percent. Perhaps this 50-fold increase in mercury vapor release partially explains why we tend to see more severe problems associated with the high copper amalgams.

As an aside to the question of mercury coming out of the filling, one might ask whether or not mercury enters the tissues of the oral cavity. Till and Maly recorded 200-300 mcg of mercury per gram of tissue in the root and bone around teeth that contained amalgam. Where amalgam was found under a gold crown, a far greater measurement was observed. In that instance, over 1200 mcg of mercury per gram of tissue was found in the tissues surrounding the tooth.(39)

To quote Catsakis and Sulica of Georgetown University, "A patient with persistent periodontitis was cured when her silver amalgam restorations were replaced. The patient decided to have only the four defective amalgam restorations on one side replaced. Soon after they were replaced with gold castings, the symptoms of periodontitis subsided on that side. The patient then decided to have the remaining restorations replaced. Shortly after the amalgam restorations were replaced, the periodontal tissue appeared healthy and remained so two years after treatment."(36)

The next question to be addressed is whether or not mercury can form a compound that is toxic. It is known that methyl mercury is more damaging than elemental mercury. It has even been stated that methyl mercury is 100 times more neurotoxic than elemental mercury.(34)

From the clinical aspect, patients appear to have more problems when they have negative electrical current in their fillings. The degree of severity of these problems does not appear to be as great when only positively charged fillings are present. I wondered if a relation exists between the presence of negative fillings and the generation of methyl mercury in the oral cavity. According to Heintze, et. al., in research done at the University of Lund at Malmo, Sweden, *Streptococcus mutans* was tested against *Clostridium cochlearium T-2* (a known methylating bacterium). Results of the tests showed that *Streptococcus mutans* has a greater ability to methylate mercury than the *Clostridium.*(33) Since *Clostridium cochlearium* has to be in a negative redox system to methylate, it is presumed that *Streptococcus mutans* may also have to have the same condition.

More severe symptoms seem to be present with negative electrical fillings in the oral cavity. It is suggested that the environment of the surface of these fillings be studied to see if the negative current actually produces a more negative redox system. If this is true, it would be more conducive to the formation of methyl mercury.

The biologic methylation of mercury is not totally dependent upon bacteria. It can follow alternative pathways and may be totally abiotic (without intervention of microbes) or may be the result of microbial metabolism. As far as potential toxicity is concerned, the neurotoxic effects of methyl mercury have already been mentioned.

Professor Claes Ramel has shown that methyl mercury is 1000 times more potent in causing genetic damage than the next most powerful agent known — Colchicine. His studies show that methyl mercury is able to produce inhibition of mitosis and chromosome breakage in the extremely low dosages of 0.1 ppm (100 mcg) or less.(34)

The references cited seem to indicate beyond a doubt that oral mercury *can* be converted to a toxic compound — deadly methyl mercury.

In addressing the next question, "Can amalgam fillings lose enough mercury to produce toxicity?", I found the following comments.

How much mercury can the body tolerate? According to Eyl, "Many scientists recommend for safety that a whole blood level of 100 ppb (parts per billion) should not be exceeded. This would correspond to a daily intake not to exceed 100 mcg."(34)

Sharma and Obersteiner (1981) state, "Mercury levels of a *few* mcg/gm severely disturb cellular function [and] growth of nerve fibers [are affected] at very much lower concentrations."(40)

I refer you again to Till's work showing mercury levels of 1200 mcg/gm of tissue under teeth containing amalgams. When Stock measured levels of over 2 mcg/M^3 in respired air, he was able to identify symptoms of mercury poisoning. Trachktenberg reported symptoms at 1 mcg. Trachktenberg was in part responsible for the Soviet Union's adoption of this standard as their maximum allowable exposure to mercury vapor. If Stock found symptoms of mercury toxicity at 2 mcg/M^3, Trachktenberg found symptoms at 1 mcg/M^3, Sharma found that a few mcg/gm would severely distrub cellular function and Eyl quotes 100 mcg per 24 hours as the maximum tolerable limit, perhaps we should look again at our potential exposures from dentistry alone. Radics found 150 mcg per 24 hours from amalgam. Gay found 49 mg/M^3 above amalgam. And Svare found 87.5 mg/M^3 in respired air.

According to these reported levels for detection of mercury toxicity, amalgam far exceeds requirements to be considered potentially detrimental.

The last question to be addressed is potentially the crux of future research. Can amalgam removal produce remission of disease symptoms? Clinical treatment that yields positive results makes the clinician enthusiastic about stating cause and effect relationships. Most of us in the clinical field are tempted to draw the conclusion that if treatment "A" renders result "B", there is a direct cause-effect relationship. This is not always the case.

In my clinical observations I have noted many health status changes after amalgam removal. It is tempting to say that mercury should be banned based upon these observations. I do realize that mercury reacts with both organic and inorganic compounds, that it affects other mineral and hormone metabolisms, that it affects enzyme activity, that its affinity for disulfide bonds lures it into multiple metabolic pathways, that it can alter both bacterial and yeast metabolism and that somewhere in this myriad lies a complexity that perhaps cannot be solved. I do feel that our clinical observations over the past eleven years suggest that attention be directed to the areas or to the specific diseases in which we have observed change. These basic areas of disease changes are set forth here for your consideration:

1. Neurological — epilepsy, multiple sclerosis, depression, suicidal tendencies

2. Cardiovascular — tachycardia, angina, unidentified chest pains

3. Collagen — scleroderma, arthritis

4. Immunological — white blood cell changes, serum protein changes

5. Allergy — food, airborne, universal reactors

If there were a common denominator of these areas, it might be said that it is reduced immunocompetence.

In summary, four questions have been addressed in regard to the feasibility of mercury being a potential problem. Answers to these questions have been provided from articles in the professional literature and from clinical observations.

BIOCHEMICAL TESTING PARAMETERS

In the clinical work we have done with mercury toxicity, we have found many biochemical tests that are altered by the removal of amalgam from the oral cavity. Because of these alterations, these tests can be con-

196

sidered diagnostic indicators. However, no one test is considered a positive diagnosis in itself. We have divided the tests into three groups based upon the depth of knowledge obtained. These three diagnostic groups are:

1. Screening
2. Clinical
3. Research

Screening procedures are those that can suggest a division between the hypersensitive patient and the mercury resistant patient. My feeling is that mercury is toxic and probably has some effect on everyone, but that some people react severely while others apparently tolerate it well. It is helpful to have simple, inexpensive tests to help identify the hypersensitive patient.

Simple screening procedures can be selected from the following list. Again, no single test is intended to confirm a positive diagnosis. A combination can suggest that a patient is relatively reactive or relatively nonreactive.

1. Body temperature
2. Electrical measurements of the fillings
3. Patient history
4. Patch test
5. Mercury vapor detection from fillings
6. Urinary excretion of mercury

Briefly, these are the interpretations we use from several years of observations. Not all patients were subjected to all tests because of their costs, the time involved and the fact that they were not all developed at the same time.

1. Body temperature: In the hypersensitive patient, there is a chance that the body temperature will be lower than normal. In most people, body temperature is lower than 98.6 degress F. upon wakening and varies during the day. We selected our readings based upon a time which could be duplicated conveniently by the patient, but which was not within one hour of awakening. Preferably these were done in the office at the same time each day. Most patients whose body temperatures were found to be within the 96 to 97 degree range said that their temperature had run low for many years. In most of the low-temperature patients, their temperature would come up to at least 98.2 degrees F. within 24 hours of removal of the last amalgam. Some patients reported readings within the 98 degree range within six hours of the final removal.

197

2. Electrical readings of the fillings: Electrical current is relative to the speed of the chemical reaction generating it. Higher electrical currents might indicate the release of more mercury vapor into the oral cavity. High and low readings do not indicate relative hypersensivity. They indicate only the relative quantity of mercury the patient is potentially receiving and the relative amount of current to which the body is being subjected.

Negative electrical readings are more frequently observed in the more serious diseases, especially those in the neurological category. The total number of fillings may or may not be directly related to the severity of the reaction. In general, the more negative fillings that are present and the greater the magnitude of the negative readings, the more severe the disease entity. We have observed occasional cases where very few negative fillings are present and yet very intense diseases are observed. These statements are based upon conditions that improved or reversed upon amalgam removal.

My clinical impression is that negative and positive readings do not correlate with equal intensity. By this I mean that a negative 5 microamp (-5) reading is not equal in devastation to a positive 5 microamp (+5) reading. A negative one (-1) reading suggests greater implications of problems than a positive fifteen (+15). The answer to this may lie in the degree of methylation that is occurring.

As a screening interpretation, the higher the current, the higher the potential for mercury vapor exposure. The greater the number of fillings, the more sources of mercury vapor. However, *current* should be more indicative of the amount of vapor than the sheer number of surfaces present. The greater the number of negative current fillings, the more potential for neurological disturbance and, from clinical observations, the greater the chance for improvement upon amalgam removal. Measurement of electrical current provides a rapid and inexpensive method of determining a patient's potential for exposure to mercury vapor.

3. Patient history: If the patient presents with numerous symptoms that have been noted to reverse in other patients after amalgam removal, the patient is more apt to respond to amalgam removal than if he were to have none of these symptoms. History provides a rapid, inexpensive index of potential hypersensitivity.

4. Patch test: In a highly hypersensitive patient, a mercury patch test will produce an exacerbation of mercury-related symptoms within 24 hours. The highly hypersensitive patient will react in an hour or less, so for this reason all patients are kept in the office for one hour after application of the patch. A reaction within one hour means that the test is over.

The patch is removed, the reaction is neutralized and usually within twenty minutes the exacerbation is over. Those patients who react within one hour are considered highly hypersensitive and could definitely be considered for amalgam removal.

Prior to placing the patch, a patient's blood pressure, pulse and temperature are recorded. At one hour, these observations are repeated. Positive reactions are suggested if the patient experiences any of the following:

a. An elevation or a drop in blood pressure of 10 points or more. In our studies we found 31 percent of the patients reacted with the described increases, while 11 percent reacted with decreases.

b. An increase or decrease of 10 points or more in pulse rate. We have noted that 25 percent of the patients tested had this kind of increase, while 13 percent demonstrated decreases.

c. Increase or decrease in body temperature of 0.5 degrees F. or more.

These observations suggest that the patient may be experiencing systemic reactions to mercury exposure.

The most significant reactions, however, are those that produce immediate symptoms such as migraine headaches, irritability or any exaggerated symptoms which have been chronic with the patient. These usually stop within a few minutes of removal of the patch and neutralization of the reaction.

5. Mercury vapor detection from fillings: This is a test similar to the electrical test in that it indicates relative exposure — not sensitivity. Two tests are usually made with one being made on the fillings as the patient presents and the other after having the patient chew gum for a set number of minutes (usually two to six). This gives an indication of vapor without oral stress and again after a simulated eating experience. We have found vapor levels in the unchallenged state to range from 0.00 mg/M^3 to 0.09 mg/M^3. After the chewing challenge, levels have been recorded from 0.01 mg/M^3 to 0.3 mg/M^3. OSHA's maximum permissible level at the present time is 0.05 mg/M^3, so it is easy to see that some amalgams can give off enormous amounts of mercury vapor relative to "safe" exposures. Some of these exposures are 600 percent greater than OSHA's maximum permissible dose for a 40 hour week. This dose hardly applies to patients who wear their fillings seven days per week.

We have combined some of these tests, and I suggest more of this be done. For instance, we have monitored a patient's EKG simultaneously with mercury vapor levels while chewing gum. In this patient, the mercury vapor increased and there were changes in the EKG during the six minute test. I do not have the expertise to evaluate the meanings of these changes, but I strongly suggest that this avenue be explored.

6. Urinary excretion of mercury: In the literature there is consistency in suggesting that high urinary excretion of mercury relates to high exposure and illness, while low levels relate to nonexposure and wellness. Almost every one of these articles includes a "however" clause. They mention something like "however, we have seen people with severe mercury toxic problems who have low levels and conversely we have seen people with high levels who were well".

While a fair amount of study has been directed toward urine, there is little agreement in interpretation of results.

The majority of the articles I have read interpret high urine mercury as a disease signal. On the other side of the coin, Kulkova as quoted by Trachktenberg states, "in patients with mercurial encephalopathy, the urinary excretion of mercury occurred *inversely* to the severity of the illness."(8)

Seifert and Neuderf in 1954 reported eight suspect and one definite mercury poisoning at very low urinary concentrations of mercury.(41)

Bidstrup says, "of the 27 persons with mercury poisoning, as a rule those with clinical evidence of mercury poisoning had a high excretion. A low excretion was also seen, however."(42)

Neal, et.al., says, "30 percent of persons with mercurialism did not have *any* mercury in their urine at all."(43)

There is variance in toxicity interpretations, too. Trachktenberg quotes opinions on the subject:

Stock suggests toxicity at 1-5 mcg/L
Trachktenberg at 1-5 mcg/L
Rutherford & Johnstone at greater than 25 mcg/L
H. Fuhner at greater than 100 mcg/L

Most U.S. laboratories I have querried consider a range of less than 20 mcg/L to be insignificant. I called the toxicology division of the Centers for Disease Control (CDC) in Atlanta, Georgia (the agency responsible for licensing and monitoring quality control in interstate laboratories). I asked them, "What do you consider the toxic limit for mercury in urine?" The answer came back, "Based on the WHO extensive study of the subject, we consider any figure in excess of 30 mcg/L to be toxic." I asked if that standard included dentistry and was informed that dentistry is a self-regulatory agency but has the responsibility of high standards.

I told him that Dr. Wilmer Eames' 1976 article in the *JADA* gave 150 mcg/L as the "allowable maximum limit in urine". In the November 1981 *ADA News,* Dr. P.L. Fan of the ADA Council on Dental Materials suggested a 500 mcg/L limit. Dr. Eames reporting in the *Journal of the Colorado Dental Assn* in 1983, moved his level up to 500 mcg/L.(44)

I asked the toxicologist spokesman from CDC, "Who has the national responsibility for setting toxic limits?" "We do," was his response.

I next asked him what his official opinion was of this rapid evolution of toxicity to 16-fold greater than that set by CDC. His answer was, *"It looks to me like an accommodation for sloppy procedures."*

In our clinical observations, we have noted that patients with severe mercury toxic reactions have *low* urinary excretions of mercury. After amalgam removal these levels *increase* in proportion to the reduction in symptom intensity. This has led us to consider that the big problem with mercury develops when the body *retains* mercury. High urinary excretion of mercury may indicate a large exposure to mercury, but disease symptoms appear to be more related to the degree of retention than to the degree of exposure.

Most hospitals or clinical laboratories consider readings of less than 20 mcg/L in the urine as normal. For this reason and for the fact that detection becomes more difficult below that level, accuracy is not paramount at very low levels. Our observations have led to the conclusion that true mercury toxicity is *retention toxicity* and that this level begins at 4 mcg/L. The relative toxicity is considered greater as the urinary excretion level approaches 0.0 mcg/L. To use mercury excretion in the urine as a screen or as a diagnostic tool, one must be able to receive data accurate to the 0.1 mcg/L at levels as low as 0.1 mcg/L. We have found significant meaning in changes of 0.5 mcg below 4 mcg/L. These changes are important in determining patient progress. Three 0.00 mcg/L levels have been observed in our practice and these patients had severe mercury toxic symptoms. As the levels of excretion increased, the patient's symptoms and other chemistries both improved.

Although it does not stand alone, urinary excretion of mercury can be used as both a screening procedure and a diagnostic test. But this is true only if the interpretation of levels as currently considered in the literature is altered. High levels may be used to indicate either increased exposure or increased excretion, whereas low levels may be looked upon as suggestive of *retention toxicity*.

Correlation and interpretation of these six tests should be considered by the doctor. The final decision as to whether or not further testing is needed rests upon the same criteria — professional judgment.

The clinical section of diagnosis encompasses those tests that meet the parameters of being both adequate and cost effective. These tests include:

1. Blood serum profile
2. Complete blood count with differential and actual platelet count
3. Hair analysis for toxicity-related metals
4. Urinary excretion of mercury

This section will cover a sampling of the type of changes seen in each area and is not intended to cover all changes in depth.

There are basic patterns in mercury toxicity which appear to become common denominators in disease manifestations. One that appears several times in apparently unassociated diseases is mercury's affinity for sulfhydryl groups. Mercury appears to have a strong affinity for sulfhydryl binding sites as well as the ability to retain this attachment once made. By its presence, it interferes with normal metabolism.

In the case of insulin, there are three sulfhydryl bonds available for mercury attachment. Our observation suggests that this attachment may happen in the mercury toxic patient. In severe cases, blood glucose levels can elevate into the diabetic range, but for the most part the elevation is slight. This elevation must be separated from those due to sugar, alcohol or caffeine. Concomitantly there will be a drop in serum cholesterol below the optimum range. Mercury can interfere with acetyl Coenzyme A activity and possibly by this mechanism reduce cholesterol production.

Dietary infractions usually produce cholesterol and glucose changes of similar magnitudes and in the same direction. When glucose goes up and cholesterol goes down, mercury toxicity is suspect. Amalgam removal procedures appear to correct these imbalances when mercury has been the cause.

Implications of this cholesterol shift are unclear at the present time. This observation is presented with the idea that some conditions of mild diabetes may not be diabetes at all, but may instead be the inability of insulin to function properly when mercury is bound to some of its three sulfhydryl binding sites.

Immunostasis to me encompasses reactions of the serum proteins and the white blood cells. A/G ratios, albumin levels and globulin levels have been examined without much meaning individually. In mercury toxicity, another ratio seems to be of more value — the Total Protein to Globulin ratio.

Jess Clifford's work in immunology gave me the idea for using this ratio. Clifford presented the concept of "globulin blocking action".(49) Mercury in the blood stream is highly reactive. For the most part, it probably unites with protein sulfhydryl groups and becomes a mercury-proteinate. In reacting against this compound, the immune system cannot perform routine immune processing functions against it, so it covers the compound with a coat of globulin. After application of the globulin coating, the offending compound becomes "transparent to the immune system". In other words, from this point forward the immune system will ignore its presence. It has been stated that higher serum globulin levels do not necessarily mean greater immune competence. Perhaps this globulin blocking action explains the reduction in the immune activity. Mercury-involved globulins may not be available for other routine immunological reactions. Clifford also described a "globulin stripping action" that releases the mercurial compound for immune processing. Immune competence must be increased for this reaction to proceed so that the mercury will not immediately reverse into its original mercury-protein compound again. Blood values of globulin are seen to drop when globulin stripping has been performed. But the value of the globulin figure itself is not helpful due to the potential movements of the Total Protein value.

To compensate for these fluctuations, the Total Protein/Globulin ratio has been applied. From clinical observations, the TP/G of 2.9-3.1 is associated with patients who show the best recoveries. As that ratio goes down, the supposition is that there is more globulin covering the mercurial compounds. A ratio below 2.6 indicates that biochemical support must be given to the patient if treatment is to be successful. Ratios below 2.1 are seen in people who respond very slowly. These people are helped by pretreatment biochemical coverage and by certain dietary considerations. One dietary problem that appears to hinder recovery from mercury toxicity is the presence of caffeine in the diet. It is suggested that the mechanism of caffeine interference involves cell membrane permeability.

Our suggestion is that the TP/G ratio can be a useful tool in suggesting immunocompetence and in monitoring treatment progress. We further suggest that ratios below 2.6 indicate more severe toxicity and the need for greater care in handling the patient.

Mercury binding to sulfhydryl groups involves another important molecule — hemoglobin. This group of reactions is commonly seen in mercury toxic patients and the results are fairly predictable. Responses in patient improvement are highly dramatic and encouraging to the patient.

Hemoglobin has four sulfhydryl binding sites. Oxygen easily attaches to these sites and just as easily releases in areas of reduced oxygen tension. Carbon dioxide rides the same hemoglobin binding sites from areas of relative CO_2 saturation back to the lungs for excretion. In people without amalgam, a balance in this reaction will usually result in a red cell count between 4.5 and 5.5 million, a hemoglobin between 13 and 15.5 grams and a hematocrit between 42 and 46 percent. Slightly lower figures may be seen in the female, and slightly higher figures may be seen in the male, but our observations suggest that the span is not as great in amalgam-free patients.

In the mercury toxic patient, severe fatigue is a frequent complaint. These patients usually sleep an average of 10 hours or more per night and either awaken fatigued or develop fatigue within a few hours of awakening. Those who have responsibilities that cannot be neglected "push" themselves to perform their daily tasks. After several trips to physicians, it is not unusual for them to be referred to psychiatrists or psychologists for treatment. Their red cell count, hemoglobin and hematocrit are usually in the high normal range. This conflicts with their complaints of fatigue.

The following theory is presented for consideration. It has many sequential areas that suggest validity, but a better test for oxygen-carrying capacity needs to be used. The tests that we have used have proved inadequate. They include oxyhemoglobin, carboxyhemoglobin, direct reticulocyte count and reticulocyte index. It is suspected that mercury attaches to one or more of hemoglobin's two sulfhydryl binding sites. In this position, mercury binds tightly — not loosely like oxygen and carbon dioxide. While bound though, oxygen and carbon dioxide cannot be transported on those sites. If only one binding site is taken by mercury, that particular hemoglobin's oxygen-carrying capacity is reduced by 25 percent.

Our theory is that, at some point, the body detects a reduction in oxygen-carrying capacity. We suggest this as an additional form of anemia. Our observation suggests that during the initial phase of mercury toxic reaction, the need for sleep is increased and the hemopoietic system undergoes a compensatory reaction. This reaction seems to produce a slight increase in red cell count (around ¼ million), a greater increase in hemoglobin (perhaps 2 gms or more) and a hemoconcentration resulting in a hemotocrit elevation of 4-8 percent.

Hematocrit is a specific level we watch, with hemoglobin secondary to it. Red cell counts move, but not to any great extent. Our observations are that upon final amalgam removal, the hematocrit will demonstrate the biggest change. It might drop from 54 percent to 44 percent within a few days. Hemoglobin and red cell count would follow suit simultaneously with an increase in patient energy levels. Sleeping habits will be altered simultaneously with the drop in cellular concentration. As much as two to three hours per night reduction in sleep requirement has been observed within a week after amalgam removal. These reactions have been so dramatic that we have looked further for explanations.

Under a modified dark field microscope, live peripheral blood cells can be videotaped before and after amalgam placement. Many red cell ghosts appear within an hour of amalgam placement. It is possible that eating and chewing gum can produce the same changes. When I began to notice large numbers of ghosts appearing I began to question just how fast the body can rebuild red blood cells to replace those nonfunctioning cells. The life expectancy of a red blood cell is reported to be 120 days. According to our pathologist consultant, Dr. David Bowerman, the body can replace all of its red cells within two to three days should it be necessary. He made one other aside comment. If this were to happen, there would be an increase in the serum enzymes alkaline phosphatase and lactic acid dehydrogenase. That comment went unregistered in my mind until I happened to notice that particular elevation in a mercury toxic patient. Checking through progress records, I noticed a strong trend toward elevation of these enzymes prior to amalgam removal.

Expansion of the theory of compensatory increase now encompasses the following suggestion. Mercury attaches to the red cell with such affinity that the body cannot remove it from the oxygen-CO_2 binding site. We propose that the body compensates for inadequate oxygen transport by hemoconcentration. Simultaneously it disassembles mercury-bound red cells and remakes new red cells with mercury-free hemoglobin. This recycling process releases alkaline phosphatase and LDH from the contaminated red cells and deposits them in the blood stream.

Our observations typically show elevations of red blood cells, Hgb, Hct, Alk Phos and LDH in the severely fatigued patient. Amalgam removal produces drops in all five levels — frequently within a week. It is quite obvious within two weeks. Alk Phos and LDH may respond slowly where toxicity is greater.

Reactions just described are those typical of the early stage mercury toxic patient. Chronic patients, we suggest, have fatigued their hemopoietic system and exhibit chronic, long-standing fatigue and low levels of red cells, Hgb and Hct. They will still have elevated Alk Phos and LDH levels. These patients require more care, slower treatment and more emphasis on nutritional principles, biochemical coverage and psychological preparations of the entire family. The consistency of these reactions relative to symptoms suggests the need to investigate the hemopoietic system for possible interrelationships with mercury toxicity.

Much to our surprise we have found that good results in the chronically ill patient sometimes produce traumatic rebounds on family members — especially the spouse. Every psychologist I have described this to has made a comment similar to, "Sure, that's to be expected."

Psychological preparation needs to be investigated and brought into focus in the treatment of the mercury toxic patient. We have found it possible to exchange a physical illness in one family member for a psychological problem in another. According to the psychologists, proper preparation of the family prior to the actual treatment of the patient could avoid this dilemma.

White blood cells lend themselves to many interpretations subsequent to amalgam removal. The initial response to amalgam placement appears to be an immune response resulting in an elevation of the white cell count. The more susceptible patients will show greater increases. Averages may be in the range of a 2500 count increase. Average white cell counts for people with amalgam are suspected to be in the range of 7500. In the absence of amalgam, the average appears to seek a level between 5000 and 5500 per cubic millimeter.

Many factors are known to alter the white cell count and the differential. Changes seen during amalgam removal are listed briefly, but with the suggestion that controlled studies be performed in this area. Our overall impression is that immunocompetence is compromised by mercury and should be a prime consideration in future studies.

We have found no way to predict which white cell population changes will occur upon amalgam placement, but we can reasonably predict what changes will occur upon amalgam removal. This is due in part to two factors. The first is that toxic reactions to mercury are individual. The second is that we have not placed amalgams in eleven years, so we have no firsthand information to examine.

Amalgam removal has produced the following changes in white blood cells. WBC's tend to optimize toward 5000 per cu. mm. Levels below that figure move upward, and levels above that figure move downward. Lymphocytes below 35 percent tend to come up, and segmented neutrophils above 55 percent tend to come down. There is another factor involved here and that is what is called actual count. Actual count is the number of cells actually present in one cubic millimeter of blood. Lymphocytes seem to have the right-of-way as white cells change. This is especially notable in the very low or very high white-cell-count patient. Lymphocytes take the lead in heading for approximately 2500 cells per cu. mm. in actual count. As the total WBC reacts, overreacts and counteracts, the *percentage* of lymphocytes may change significantly, but the actual count will tend strongly to seek 2500 at the expense of the other cells. Within the lymphocyte population, the T-lymphs seem to increase rapidly after amalgam removal.

Monocytes in a normal distribution are usually considered acceptable and not out of place at levels of 1-3 percent. In treating the mercury toxic patient, levels in excess of 6 percent are occasionally noted. No matter what level is found initially, it is not uncommon to see a reduction to 0 in monocytes after the patient is amalgam free. We feel that this lends itself to a reevaluation of the presence of monocytes in the "normal" patient.

Basophils occasionally appear at levels of 1-3 percent and these usually drop to 0 within a short period of time after amalgam removal. There is some discussion as to whether or not Basophils are involved with toxic reactions. Their behavior after amalgam removal suggests that they may play a role in heavy metal toxicity.

Eosinophils normally elevate during allergic reactions. Allergies were not suspected of being involved with mercury reactions until about 1980, so we don't have long-term observations on the behavior patterns of eosinophils as related to allergy and mercury. Short-term behavior is reasonably consistent. Not everyone with amalgam has allergies, but when a person does have allergic reactions (to airborne as well as to food substances), allergy can be reflected in eosinophil counts. The usual reaction is to see the eosinophil count drop to about one fourth of its original level after amalgam removal. Some cases we have seen have been outstanding, and amalgam removal has evidenced a reduction to 0-2 percent eosinophil count.

The most severe allergy case we have seen was an M.D. who had records showing a maximum eosinophil count of 64 percent a few months before we saw him. A CBC was done the day amalgam removal procedures were started. It showed 46 percent Eos. Within the same week and only part way through the amalgam removal procedures, another CBC was run. Due to the difference in eosinophils, four slides were prepared and sent to four hospitals for differential counts. My technician and the four hospitals all came up with the same count — Eos 2 percent.

Symptoms markedly changed within that week. From being what allergists term a "universal reactor" for several years, he could eat almost any food and could be around people and odors he had not tolerated in several years. In his case, there was a strong suggested link between allergies, eosinophils and amalgam.

In many patients, Bands react immediately to amalgam removal. Percentage-wise this occurs about half of the time. When the reaction does take place, it is reasonably consistent. Bands are immature cells and are not found in the blood of truly healthy, unchallenged people. Upon amalgam removal, Bands appear at a level of around 4 percent if none were present initially. If several percent were there, the count will tend to increase by 3-4 percent. This reaction takes place within a short time and Bands may continue at this level for up to six weeks. After this time, the level tends to drop to 0.

Since white cell responses are reflective of immune challenge, I suggest that hematology could play a big role in determining the role of amalgam in human immunocompetence. I would also suggest that the changes in white cells which are produced by amalgam removal should discourage the use of amalgam in human subjects.

Hair analysis has received a moderate amount of press in the last few years — some positive, some negative. The arguments seem to center around a lack of identical results from different laboratories and a lack of understanding of interpretation. Having been in the industry involving blood and hormones, hair and many other analyses, I feel that I can take a moderated view of the subject.

Hair metal values frequently do not start until the sixth decimal down from one gram. At this level, a difference between a "1" and a "2" should possibly be considered in light of its magnitude. To call this a 100 percent difference may be implying things that are not true. One thing that is not usually considered is that conventional medical laboratories running routine tests vary in significant magnitudes. These not being new methods of testing, few people test one lab against another. The only laboratories that are monitored by an outside agency are those with an interstate license. They are fewer than 10 percent of all laboratories. All hair analysis laboratories are under interstate license monitoring by the Centers for Disease Control.

In Colorado, I sent a split sample of serum to two different hospitals for cholesterol testing. One hospital reported 150 mg percent, while the other reported over 200 mg percent. At that time the total normal range was 150 mg percent to 300 mg percent. I also sent a split sample to the *same* hospital. Afterwards I found that they were labeled samples number 23 and 24, so I assumed they were run at approximately the same time. The same sample, at the same hospital, run at the same time gave readings of 150 mg percent and 300 mg percent. Those are the outer borders of the range and certainly could be significant if considered as part of the diagnosis of a heart patient.

Interpretation in the field of mineral analysis needs more investigation because of its newness. Many changes occur that are not readily apparent, so suggestions are made. Last week I saw a newspaper article on hair analysis suggesting that cobalt levels might be reflective of vitamin B-12 levels because cobalt is part of the B-12 reaction. I have simultaneously tested vitamin B-12 and hair cobalt in the same patients. I have not found anything I personally would consider reflective of biological similarity.

Over the past sixteen years, I have seen over 25,000 hair analyses in conjunction with other biological parameters (blood, CBC, urine, hormones, vitamins) and have drawn conclusions as to which minerals are reflective of biological conditions and which are not.

In the mercury-toxic patient we have identified five minerals that suggest toxicity. The first three must appear as a triad (calcium, manganese and mercury). Then the next two (zinc and potassium) will appear in accordance with the severity of the reaction. If these five minerals appear out of bounds in a random order, we do not consider them involved in mercury toxicity.

In the mercury-toxic patient, all three elements of the triad can be either excessive or deficient. However, none will be within the accepted range. The most serious combination is high calcium, low manganese and low mercury. It occurs both "most often" and in the "most difficult to correct" cases. There is a possibility of interreactions between sialic acid, calcium and mercury which in turn could lead to decreased cellular permeability. Again, further investigation. . . .

As the case intensifies in disease-type responses, a lowering of the zinc level usually appears. In the most severe cases — the neurological cases — the potassium will drop into the less than 10 ppm range.

As a general observation, the more divergent the patient values from our norm and the greater the number of imbalances (from three to five), the more severe the symptoms.

Another observation is that disease intensity is generally related to the divergence from the norm of each individual mineral. A patient with a calcium level of 4000 ppm would be expected to exhibit more symptoms than one with 2000 ppm (400 to 600 being the anticipated range).

Urine mercury levels have already been discussed under screening procedures. It is highly significant as a diagnostic method because of its ability to indicate retention toxicity. From the practical standpoint, this level gives an indication of how severe the patient's condition is and how quickly he can be expected to respond. As urinary excretion drops below 4 mcg/L, one can expect more severe symptoms and slower responses. Monitoring of the urinary excretion of mercury can also be useful in determining patient progress.

These four testing parameters have been useful in determining relative toxicity of patients and have provided a system of monitoring that indicates progress or the lack of progress. For more in-depth analysis of systemic reactions, the following tests are suggested on the basis of observation. Experience and lack of professional assistance in interpretation has handicapped the use of these tests for practical diagnostic procedures. But that should not minimize the importance of investigation into these areas.

Research is a category that expands continually. Tests have been run where it was suspected that changes could be found. Since none of our patients want amalgam replaced just for science, we thought it best to have the test records completed and wait for future funding to hire experts for interpretation. The percentage of change sounds signficant, but I have no way of confirming this at this time.

Electrocardiogram measurements sometimes change by 200 to 300 percent after amalgam removal. Electroencephalograms have transformed from abnormal to normal in a seizure patient who became seizure-free after amalgam removal. Aluminum (as in temporary crowns) when placed in a mouth containing amalgam can cause brain Alpha waves to increase by 1000 percent.

Are these changes due to chemical toxicity, due to alteration of electrical output of the fillings or due to a combination of both? In some cases, the electrical current generated in the fillings (actually in reasonable proximity to the brain) are several fold greater than the 7-9 nanoamperes of current the brain generates during normal function. Since initial control of heart rhythm is within the brain, does the malfunction of one contribute to the malfunction of the other? I have two questions. First I ask, are these changes significant? And second, should dentistry be placing materials that could potentially alter brain and cardiac function?

These are serious questions that I feel should be addressed by the researchers at the National Institutes of Health. They are obviously beyond the scope of conventional dental research.

A University of Colorado PhD devised a psychological test for our patients. His initial observation was that "people process thought differently with amalgam in their mouths than without." He found a marked increase in ability to cope as one of the most frequent changes.

Lack of funding has prevented us from getting more in-depth interpretations, but we have many test results available for completion and evaluation. Other psychologists have suggested the use of standard questionnaires with standardized interpretations. However, they have indicated that the presence of mercury might alter the interpretations. Initial observation of changes would probably be necessary just to determine what areas are worthy of investigation.

Fundus photography has provided a new method of monitoring changes in the retina of the eye. Eye specialists have noted a relationship between myopia, cataracts and mercury exposures for several years. Some colleges are now interested in researching these avenues.

There is a black streak which appears around the optic disc in the retinas of some people. It has been interpreted for years by physicians to be an artifact produced in the myopic eye due to its physical elongation. Stretching of the retina was thought to produce thinning in this area and what was visualized was thought to be the underlying epithelium showing through the stretched retina. It is challenging to this theory to note that these streaks occur only in people with amalgam in their mouths. It is further suggestive of the need for new interpretation when one finds that these black areas tend to disappear after amalgam removal. The slide presentation will demonstrate these changes.

On or about 400 BC, Hippocrates recommended, "The physician will examine to see whether one side (of the patient) is hotter than the other. Should one part of the body be hotter or colder than the rest, disease is present in that part."(46)

This gives us cause to wonder about the body temperature changes that occur after amalgam removal. Good use has been made of that knowledge, although it was not until the 19th century that a scientific understanding was uncovered. On April 24, 1800, William Herschel, who was King George III's Astronomer Royal, announced that he had discovered invisible rays in the spectrum of the sun. He called them infrared.(47) Herschel, Stefan and Boltzmann discovered that all solid materials in the environment emit infrared radiation. As a result of their research, Stefan and Boltzmann formulated the Stefan-Boltzmann Law. This law states that solid bodies will radiate energy in the form of electromagnetic waves at a rate proportional to the fourth power of the temperature.(45)

This law is the basis upon which thermography was developed. Sensitive infrared cameras can now detect changes in body temperature of 0.1 degree C. Oncologists make use of this noninvasive diagnostic method because a malignant tumor may have a temperature one or more degrees

Centigrade above the surrounding tissues. Mammography has been its primary use in recent years.

Neurologists enjoy thermography for its noninvasive qualities plus the additional information it offers. X-rays show bone and intracranial substances, the electroencephalogram is good for determining physiological integrity of the brain and computer assisted tomography (CAT scan) shows relative density of soft tissues. Thermography offers something none of these offer — the relative blood supply to regions of the skull and brain.

It is generally accepted that the thermographic pattern of the head remains somewhat constant. It has been referred to as the fingerprint. Recently, Dr. Bill Dudley, president of the International Thermographic Society, called to tell us of the enormous changes that occur in the head after amalgam removal. In a patient with ALS, the circulation to the brain doubled as amalgams were removed. On the videotape presentation, a portion of the diagnostic film will be shown visualizing changes that are quite obvious even to the untrained eye.

Circulation to the brain could be a critical issue to some patients. If indeed, amalgam (either through electrical current or toxicity of methyl mercury) is responsible for interference with head and neck circulation, a great deal of effort should be put into investigations immediately. None of us really want to damage our patients.

Specific gravity of the urine is neither difficult nor expensive but does deserve attention because of its relationship to posterior pituitary activity. It has been suggested that emotional stability is influenced by posterior pituitary activity. Measurements of specific gravity changes should probably be done simultaneously with psychological testing to determine if correlations really exist between emotional health, posterior pituitary activity and amalgam.

One of the research tools I particularly enjoy is cell morphology as viewed under Hoffman contrast microscopy. Hoffman contrast offers many advantages over bright field microscopy in the area of metal toxicity. Hoffman gives all the contrast without the bloom of bright field. With part of the light source coming from the side of the slide, a 3-D effect similar to Numarsky optics is seen. For metal toxicity, Hoffman appears to be superior to Numarsky optics because the latter does not produce spectral separations. The differences in color separation give Hoffman better detail of cytoplasmic and nuclear details.

It has been observed that when a patient is experiencing metal toxicity, there is an elevation of Haloed Bodies in the Monocytes. Haloed Bodies are secondary lysosomal structures that are not seen under bright field, but can be discerned under Hoffman contrast.(49) These structures reduce in number fairly quickly during the first week after amalgam removal and then a further, gradual reduction seems to take place over the ensuing months.

Another interesting pattern to follow is the reduction of Excrescences from the nucleus after amalgam removal. The origin of an Excresence (a whip-like appendage extruding from the nuclear membrane) is believed to be that it is literally pulled out by the remains of the centriole-centrisome system under a metabolic dysfunction. The centriole-centrisome systems are attachments to the lobes of the nucleus and which may be used for massage and locomotion of the nucleus under certain processes.(49)

In cases of metal toxicity, the percentage of polymorphonuclear leukocytes (PMN) with excrescent activity can reach as high as 15-17 percent. Reduction usually occurs after amalgam removal.

Mercury toxicity has been known for years to produce multilobular PMN's in acute exposures. Many times PMN's with four or more lobes can be seen in the mercury toxic patient. There is also an imbalance favoring the two-lobed PMN's (Bifeds). After amalgam removal, the three-lobed PMN's (Trifeds) dominate the scene with almost all four-lobed PMN's disappearing. A simultaneous reduction of Bifeds can also be noted. These counts require special attention because in a routine differential, Bifeds, Trifeds and Fourfeds are usually lumped together under the heading of Segs or Segmented Neutrophils.

As mentioned earlier, amalgam removal can produce an increase in T-lymphs and a simultaneous decrease in B-lymphs. Under Hoffman contrast it is notable that not only does the percentage change, but the new T-lymph population is predominately composed of the small lymphs (6-9 microns), while less medium and large lymphs are seen.

Hoffman contrast offers one more useful observation that is not available under bright field. Under Hoffman, cytoplasms can be separated into four types, based upon stippling or granulation. After amalgam removal, cytoplasmic granulation tends to revert to the fine, smooth, light staining of Type I.

Normal platelet counts range from 150,000 to 400,000 depending upon the laboratory. We have noted that mercury toxic patients tend toward the extremes of the range. Most exhibit higher counts, but a small percentage will exhibit very low counts. Platelets tend to be a little larger in mercury toxicity and tend to form clumps. After amalgam removal, we have observed the high readings coming down and the low readings coming up. They tend to seek a level between 225,000 and 250,000, often by the two week follow-up chemistry.

Treatment planning presented here is based upon the practical diagnostic tests. In actual practice, other parameters may be added if deemed necessary.

Experience has taught us that success and failure can be affected during the treatment phase. Recovery from mercury toxicity is not simply a matter of removing amalgam. The body must be able to eliminate the stored mercury also.

Our current treatment involves solving two very important, different but intertwining problems. One is chemical toxicity and the other is electrical interference with nerve impulse transmission. Both are important and must be confronted if the patient is to recover.

Sad experience has taught us that amalgam removal without observing certain principles can result in two unpleasant events. One is an exacerbation of the patient's symptoms and the other is a suspension of improvement. Both undesirable results can be generated by removing fillings with positive electrical current first while leaving those with negative current behind. In order to have the best chance for success we have observed that sequential removal of amalgams is essential. Sequential removal involves removing fillings with the highest negative current first, followed by the lower negatives. The next to be removed are the high positive fillings and finally the low positives. This can be done by quadrants and does not have to be done by individual fillings.

Even if a quadrant contains both high positive and negative current fillings, the positives can be removed along with the negatives as long as the negative in that arch is the highest negative reading in the mouth.

There is some suggestion that high copper amalgams may tend to be negative more often than conventional amalgams, but this is not definite. It has been observed that when a high negative-high copper amalgam exists in a patient with neurological disorders, the chances of successful treatment are greatly reduced. Recovery is slow and exacerbations are set off easily.

Rarely does a gold crown exhibit negative current. We have only recorded two in over 1000 tests. Nonprecious crowns do give negative readings. I do not have figures on this because our patients do not often have nickel crowns in their mouths. An educated guess would place the figure at around one-third being negative and two-thirds being positive. When negative crowns are found, it is common to find neurological problems associated with them. As with amalgam, removal of the negative crowns produces improvement in symptoms and chemistries within a few days or weeks. We have noted similar improvements in patients who have nickel in their mouths with no amalgam present. This may suggest that metal toxicity can occur with nickel as well as with mercury.

There are several methods readily available for ridding the body of toxic metals. Most of these involve a process called chelation. Three drugs that are in common usage are British Anti-Lewisite (BAL), EDTA and Penicillamine. All three have severe side effects and are considered undesirable for this reason.

Biochemical coverage prior to amalgam removal seems to be as important as sequential removal. If this is started 48 hours or more prior to amalgam removal procedures, chances for improvement are increased. If they are not initiated, chances for improvement are slight. Biochemical coverage is determined by the blood chemistry, hair analysis, CBC, urinary excretion and other tests where available.

Biochemical coverage should provide aid in the areas of:

1. increasing selective permeability of the cell membrane
2. encouraging the cells to excrete mercury
3. globulin stripping
4. providing a ligand for mercury for excretory transport
5. reducing hormonal imbalances

In more severe cases, especially those involving negative electrical current and neurological disorders, the use of Protamine Zinc Insulin reduces the exacerbations common to removal of high negative current fillings. It is suggested that this help is provided by stabilizing the parasympathetic division of the autonomic nervous system.

Basic biochemical coverage is provided by specific minerals, vitamins C, A and E, digestive enzymes, iodine, thyroid hormone and posterior pituitary hormone. These are selected on the basis of need shown in the individual patient's chemistries.

Follow-up chemistries provide information as to the length of time for treatment and alterations in dosage that might be required. If the initial treatment is not successful, we look to the area of *Candida albicans*. We have recently found a relationship between the presence of amalgam and the increase in symptoms of *Candida albicans*. Since the symptoms of *Candida* and those of mercury toxicity overlap in so many areas, the possibility of both being involved should always be considered.

Perhaps it would be worthwhile to explore our preliminary observations on the subject of *Candida*. There appears to be a connection between the presence of amalgam and the body's ability to cope with the yeast, *Candida albicans*. *Candida* is considered normal flora, but when the body's immune mechanisms are impaired, *Candida* can increase until it produces disease-type symptoms. Since this is a new concept, we do not have large numbers of patients to draw from, but those we do have seem to suggest the following hypothesis.

It appears that there may be a cohabitation of factors that produce an ecosystem conducive to the development of both problems. Two factors seem to stand out in examining conditions of similarity. *Candida* can live under negative redox conditions. Methylation of mercury by *Streptococcus mutans* proceeds better under negative redox conditions. By-products of both reactions may feed each other and create an alternative metabolic pathway for *Candida*. This alternative metabolic pathway may bypass the normal route involving actions blocked by Nystatin thereby rendering its pharmacologic action ineffective.(50) Removal of the methylating system reestablishes the usual metabolic pathway for *Candida*, perhaps explaining the improvement in Candidiasis observed after amalgam removal.

Observations of the systemic reactions of mercury, especially with the potential for methyl mercury formation in the mouth, lead one to challenge the biocompatibility of amalgam as a dental restorative material.

CONCLUSION

Our conclusions, based on clinical studies and observations, are that we may have been looking at the wrong area for toxicity. In the past, the question has been, "Does mercury come out of the filling or not?" I believe there is adequate material through vapor studies and analysis of dated amalgams to substantiate that it does.

From this point, our thinking has previously been directed toward elemental mercury. New evidence suggests that we should have been studying methyl mercury. With the proximity of *Streptococcus mutans* to mercury on the surface of amalgam, a whole new picture evolves. It is one that presents our foe, methyl mercury, as 100 times more neurotoxic than elemental mercury. We see methyl mercury as 1000 times more capable of genetic damage than the second most harmful substance known — Colchicine. This suggests that we should actually be looking at the safety limits of 0.05 mcg/M^3 divided by 100 or divided by 1000.

Negative electrical current is practically newborn in our systems of analysis. Clinical observation suggests that far more toxicity is exhibited

216

when negative current is present. Our tentative suggestion is that negative electrical current may be a factor in the generation of methyl mercury. Negative electrical current may help produce a chemical negative redox system highly compatible with the methylation of mercury by *Streptococcus mutans*. If this it true, then we suggest that mercury be eliminated as a dental restorative material.

REFERENCES

1. Emory, S., *Actualizations,* Doubleday & Co., 1977.

2. Peters, T.J., Waterman, R.H., *In Search of Excellence,* Warner Books, 1982.

3. *JAMA,* Vol 243, March, 1980.

4. Editorial, *JADA* Vol 82, Mar, 1971.

5. Chandler, H.H., Rupp, H.W., Paffenbarger, G.C., Poor mercury hygiene from ultrasonic amalgam condensation, *JADA* Vol 82, No 3, March, 1971.

6. Patrick, J.J.R., Oral electricity and new departure, *D. Cosmos,* 22:543, Oct, 1880.

7. Espevik, S., *Ann. Rev. Mater. Sci.* 7, 1977, p.55.

8. Trachktenberg, I.M., *Chronic Effects of Mercury on Organisms,* DEW Publication No. (NIH) 74-473, 1974.

9. Wranglen, G., Berendson, J., Electrochemical aspects of corrosion processes in the oral cavity with special reference to amalgam fillings, R. Inst. Technol Ser. on corrosion and surface protection of metals.

10. Wranglen, G., Metallers Korrosion och Ytskydd, Almgvist & Wiksell, Stockholm 1967, p.47.

11. Wranglen, G., *Corr. Sci.* Vol 9, 1969, p.585.

12. Wranglen, G., *Corr. Sci,* Vol 14, 1974, p.331.

13. Wranglen, G., Localized Corrosion, NACE-3, Houston 1974, p.462.

14. Wranglen, G., Sulfide Inclusion in Steel, ASM-6, Metals Park 1975, p. 361.

15. Berendson, J., & Wranglen, G., *Corr. Sci,* Vol 20, 1980, p. 937.

16. Tuccillo, J.J., & Neilsen, J.P., *J. Pros. Dent.* 31, 1974, p.285.

17. Wranglen, G., & Berendson, J., Electrochemical aspects of corrosion processes in the oral cavity with special reference to amalgam fillings, Royal Inst. Technol., Corrosion and surface protection of metals.

18. Frykholm, K.O., Hedegard. B., *Svensk Tandiakartidskrift 61*, 1968, p. 435.

19. Mumford, J.M., Electrolytic action in the mouth and its relationship to pain, *J. Dent. Res.* 636, 1957.

20. Wranglen, G., personal communication with Jaroslav Pleva, Sept 22, 1982.

21. Bergman, M., Ginstrup, O., *Acta Odont. Scand.* 33, 1975, p.199.

22. Tani, G., Zucchi, F., *Minerva Stomatol* 16, 1967, p.710.

23. Montyla, D.G., Wright, O.D., Mercury toxicity in the dental office: a neglected problem, *JADA* Vol 92, No. 6, June 1976.

24. Koos, Longo, Pregnancy, *Pediatrics*, Vol. 64, No. 5, Nov 1979.

25. Eames, W.B., et.al., The mercury enigma in dentistry, *JADA* Vol 92, No. 6, June 1976.

26. Brecht-Bergen, N., *Zeitschr. Elektroch.* 39, 1933, p.927.

27. Stock, A., Die Chronisch Quecksilber and Amalgam vergiftung, Zahnorztl, *Rumdschau* 48, 1939, p.403.

28. Gay, D.D., Cox, R.D., and Reinhard, J.W.,: Chewing releases mercury from fillings, *Lancet*, May 5, 1979, p.985.

29. Svare, C.W., et.al. The effect of dental amalgams on mercury levels in expired air, *J. Dental Res.* 50, Sept 1981.

30. Hanson, M., Amalgam — Hazards in your teeth, *J. Orthomol, Psych.* Vol 12, No. 3, Sept 1983.

31. Pleva, J., Mercury poisoning from dental amalgam, *J. Orthomol. Psych.* Vol 12, No. 3, Sept 1983.

32. Radics, J., et.al., Die kristallinin kompenenten der silberamalgam untersuchungen mit der elektronischen rontgenmikrosorde, *Zahuarzfl Welf* 79, 1031, 1970.

33. Heintze, M., et.al., Methylation of mercury from dental amalgam and mercuric chloride by oral streptococci in vitro., Scand. J. Dent. Res. 9, 1983, 150-2.

34. Eyl, T.B., Methyl mercury poisoning in fish and human beings, *Modern Med.*, Vol. 38, Nov, 1970.

35. Summers, A.O., Silver, S., Microbial transformations of metals. *Ann. Rev. Microbiol.* 1978; 32:637-672.

36. Catsakis, L.J., Sulica, V.I., Allergy to silver amalgams, *Oral Surg* 46: 371-375, Sept 1978.

37. Barkowski, *North Carolina Dent J.*, Spring 1979.

38. Mayhall, C.W., Letter to Editor, *JADA* Vol 82, No. 6, June 1971.

39. Till, T., Maly, K.,: Zum Nachweis der Lyse von Hg aus Silberamalgam von Zahnfullungen, *Der Praktische Arzt*, 1042, Sept, 1978.

40. Sharmo, R.P., Obersteiner, E.J.,: Metals and neurotoxic effects: cytotoxicity of selected metallic compounds on chick ganglia cultures, *J. Comp. Pathol*, 91, 235, 1981.

41. Seifert, P. and Neudert, H., Zur Frage der gewerblichen Quecksilber-Vergiftung, *Zbl. Arbeitsmed*, 4, 129, 1954.

42. Bidstrup, P.L., et. al., Chronic mercury poisoning in men repairing direct-circuit meters, *Lancet*, 251, 856, 1951.

43. Neal, P.A., Jones, R., Chronic mercurialism in the hatter's fur-cutting industry, *JAMA*, 110, 337, 1938.

44. Eames, W.B., Mercomania strikes again, *J. Colo Dent Assn.* Vol 62, No. 3, Nov-Dec, 1983, p.3.

45. Uematsu, S., *Medical Thermography, Theory and Clinical Applications* Brentwood Pub Corp., 1976.

46. Chadwick, J., Mann, W.M., *Hippocrates — Medical works*, Oxford: Blackwell, 1950.

47. Herschel, W., Investigations of the powers of the prismatic colours to heat and illuminate objects. *Phil. Trans. Roy. Soc.* 90:255-92, 1800.

48. Brune, D., et.al., Gastrointestinal and in vitro release of copper, cadmium, indium, mercury and zinc from conventional and copper-rich amalgams. *Scand. J. Dental. Res.*, 1983,; 91:66-71.

49. Clifford, W.J., Harper, H.W., The immunostatus differential, *J. Internat'l Acad. Prev. Med.*, Vol. 6, No. 1, 1979.

50. Clifford, W.J., personal communication.

The following thirteen pages were included in a press kit and given to members of the media prior to an unprecedented press conference following the workshop. Read it carefully and then compare it to the next set of recommendations.

RECOMMENDATIONS

Workshop on the Biocompatibility of Metals in Dentistry

July 11-13, 1984

This gathering was sponsored by the National Institute of Dental Research and hosted by the American Dental Association. The workshop was convened in order to accomplish two basic objectives:

1. To review what is currently known from existing scientific evidence and literature about the various metals used in dentistry; and
2. To pinpoint areas of interest or concern that may warrant further research, in the opinion of the workshop as a whole.

More than 200 dental researchers, practicing dentists and physicians from around the world participated in this workshop. Over the past three days, 11 presentations were made on a wide range of topics related to the biocompatability of dental metals. It was from these presentations and the discussions that ensued that we developed the recommendations we are announcing here today.

With the public interest in mind, the dental profession is continually reviewing and evaluating the materials used in treating patients. This workshop stands as part of that on-going effort to ensure that the materials dentists use are of the highest quality and that they are compatable with oral and general health.

The recommendations from this workshop are offered to identify for the dental research community those areas of research the workshop believes should be further investigated.

Metals are used in dentistry in a variety of ways. Dentures, orthodontic braces, crowns and caps and dental amalgam fillings all contain metals of various types. Data was presented at this workshop on a number of dental metals. Some of those most commonly used in dentistry include gold, nickel, tin, copper, silver, and mercury.

In recent years, questions have been raised on the use of mercury in dental amalgam fillings — what most people know as the silver fillings dentists use to restore teeth damaged by tooth decay.

These questions have been raised within the dental profession and the general public.

In light of public and professional concerns on this issue, it was decided that the workshop's recommendations pertaining to mercury and dental amalgam should be announced immediately. A full report of the workshop proceedings and recommendations will be published as soon as possible in the *Journal of the American Dental Association.*

Regarding the use of dental amalgam as an effective restorative material, the two key questions are these:

1. Is there sufficient documented evidence to recommend discontinuing the use of dental amalgam in dental practice?

2. Is there sufficient documented evidence to recommend that patients with dental amalgam in their mouths have it removed?

Based on the information presented and evaluated during the three days of this workshop, the answer to the first question is an unequivocal no. There is not sufficient documented evidence to recommend discontinuing the use of dental amalgam.

The answer to the second question is also no, with one qualification.

In the judgement of the workshop as a whole, dental amalgam is a safe and effective restorative material for the majority of Americans.

There is, however, documented evidence that a small percentage of the population is hypersensitive to mercury. These individuals, exhibiting a true allergic reaction to the metal, can be identified through a combination of medical history review and testing.

The removal of dental amalgam can only be recommended in those patients who are proven to be allergic to mercury.

To assist in identifying these patients, the workshop recommends:

1. Immediate initiation of a survey to assess the prevalence of mercury allergy in the United States population.

2. Initiation of studies to develop more definitive tests for detecting cases of hypersensitivity or allergy to metals used in dentistry; and

3. Initiation of studies to accurately assess body levels of mercury that may result from dental amalgam.

As a result of recent technological developments, we are now able to measure extremely small amounts of mercury released from dental amalgams in the form of mercury vapor.

Evidence was presented to the workshop showing that mercury vapor is released from the surface of dental amalgams. It was particularly evident that this release occurs at least primarily during chewing.

It is logical that some of this mercury vapor released from dental fillings is inhaled and absorbed into the blood stream.

It should be emphasized, however, that the amount of mercury eminating from dental fillings is extremely small. It should be noted, too, that mercury is introduced to the human system through a variety of other sources — including the air we breathe, the foods we eat, the water we drink and through the bad habit some of us have called smoking.

The mercury we receive each day from these nondental sources far exceeds the minuscule amount released from dental fillings.

No documented evidence was presented to the workshop proving that this low level release of mercury from dental amalgams constitutes a health risk. Nevertheless, we believe it is our responsibility as health professionals to thoroughly review all aspects of this issue.

To do so, the workshop issues the following specific recommendations:

1. An assessment should be made of mercury loss from chewing on dental amalgams of different alloy composition.

2. Biological sampling procedures should be investigated to determine a definitive means of estimating the body burden of mercury.

3. Studies are encouraged to determine whether a relationship exists between maternal exposure to mercury and effects on the fetus; and

4. Research should be initiated to determine whether the effects of mercury on T-lymphocytes, a white blood cell, may be a means of early detection of mercury toxicity.

In addition to these research recommendations, the workshop also pinpointed certain positive actions that practicing dentists should implement.

First, the workshop recommends that dentists should include in all patient records, documentation on individuals sensitive to mercury and all materials used in dentistry.

Second, all practitioners are encouraged to review the symptoms of metal exposure.

And *third,* practitioners are encouraged to report all case histories of reactions to, or effects from, biomaterials to the American Dental Association.

This set of recommendations was sent to us after the workshop. Notice the changes as seen from the first set which was completed prior to our presentation.

BIOCOMPATIBILITY OF METALS IN DENTISTRY

SUMMARY

Metals are routinely used in dentistry in a variety of applications. These include the use of metals in fabrication of prosthetic appliances, orthodontic bands, temporary and permanent crowns, and in direct restoration of teeth. The metals most commonly used in dentistry include gold, nickel, cobalt, chromium, tin, aluminum, titanium, iron, palladium, platinum, copper, silver, vanadium and mercury. These metals have been used successfully in dentistry for a number of years. However, improvements in the sensitivity of evaluating dental materials raises questions in the clinical and research communities regarding their safety and efficacy. It is incumbent upon the dental profession to continually review and assess the dental materials used in treating patients to ensure that these materials are of the highest quality and are compatible with oral tissue and general health.

This workshop has examined the use of metals in dentistry from several perspectives. These include the potential for their toxicity in living systems, their allergic potential, their carcinogenic potential, clinical experience with metals, and the current status of the development of alternative materials for use in restorative procedures.

Following is a summary of the information presented on these subjects by the workshop participants. In addition, recommendations for future research and clinical implementation in the area of the biocompatibility of metals in dentistry are presented.

NICKEL
Nickel is commonly used in alloys in prosthetic devices. These devices are composed of alloys of nickel and chromium or cobalt, with nickel content as high as 81 percent. Their use is increasing as an alternative for materials containing gold and other metals. It is important to continue to assess the safety of the use of nickel in dental applications.

Nickel has been implicated as a toxic material in several non-dental applications. Air-borne exposure to nickel in dusts has been related to its potential to induce carcinogenesis in nasal and lung tissue. The type of nickel compounds in the dental environment should be identified and quantified to determine their carcinogenic potential. In addition, nickel is

226

a common sensitizer. Contact with nickel-containing jewelry, buttons, zippers and clasps on clothing induces sensitization. The prevalence is an estimated 10 percent in women and less than 1 percent in men. Allergic reactions to nickel can be manifested both locally and systemically from contact with the skin. Reactions to nickel by the mucous membranes have been reported.

When a nickel allergy is suspected, it is possible to verify the sensitivity through patch testing. Patch testing on the skin in conjunction with a history and/or clinical symptoms of nickel allergy is an acceptable predictor of sensitivity. The high frequency of both false-positive and false-negative tests suggests the need for verification. Routine patch testing of patients for nickel sensitivity, however, it not recommended. When clinical symptoms cause a dentist to suspect an allergy to nickel, the patient should be screened via patch testing by a professional trained in the administration and interpretation of the tests. Referral to allergists or dermatologists who specialize in this testing is recommended.

BERYLLIUM
Base-metal alloys used in constructing prosthetic devices contain beryllium at levels from 0.48 percent to 1.89 percent. Although toxicity to beryllium has been reported from occupational exposure in other industrial areas, no cases have been reported from a contact with dental materials containing beryllium. Lung cancer has been reported in occupationally-exposed workers, including dental laboratory technicians. However, the study on dental laboratory technicians could not isolate beryllium as the carcinogen. Additionally, it is possible to reduce the exposure of technicians to zero with proper ventilation of working zones. Due to the absence of reports of toxicity and limited exposure, current base-metal alloys containing beryllium are not presently considered to be a risk for dental patients.

COBALT
Cobalt is a constituent of base-metal alloys and has been reported to be capable of inducing sensitization. The prevalence of individuals allergic to cobalt is estimated to be less than 1 percent and appears to be isolated to females. Contact sensitivity has been diagnosed by patch testing. When a history and/or clinical symptoms suggest a potential allergy to an alloy containing cobalt, additional testing is necessary to verify that the allergy is related to cobalt.

CHROMIUM
Base-metal alloys which contain nickel and cobalt also commonly contain chromium. Certain forms of chromium have been associated with lung cancer in industrial exposures. However, carcinogenesis related to dental and medical applications has not been reported. Chromium has been

reported to sensitize individuals and to produce a chronic dermatitis. The sensitivity is due to contact with chromate salts which result from the corrosion of such alloys. The dermatitis produced in individuals sensitive to chromium may continue for a number of years and in some cases may result in a serious cosmetic problem. Reports of allergy to chromium are rare. Patch testing may identify a chromium-sensitive patient, but there is a risk in testing patients because of the potential for sensitizing them through patch testing. Chromium allergy related to contact in the mouth is reported to be rare.

GOLD
Sensitization from contact with gold is reported to be extremely rare. Most patients who report allergy to gold are usually sensitive to nickel, cobalt, or chromium as components of jewelry that may be goldplated. Allergy to gold is not considered to be a problem in dentistry.

MERCURY
Considerable interest has been focused recently on the possible effects of mercury vapor released from the surfaces of dental amalgam. New technologies which permit detection of very low levels of mercury in the air and body tissues have raised questions as to whether the small levels of mercury released from amalgam surfaces can pose a possible risk for patients with amalgam restorations.

Studies have demonstrated that patients are exposed to mercury vapor when amalgams are placed as a restoration, when existing amalgams are removed, and during chewing. Some studies suggest that blood levels of mercury are elevated in patients during these procedures and that the levels are correlated with the number of amalgams and the occluding surface area. Other studies have demonstrated no difference in blood levels in patients with and without amalgam restorations. Additional studies in this area are required to more accurately assess the possible risk to patients.

Health hazards of blood mercury levels associated with dental amalgams have not been documented. It is difficult, therefore, to interpret the relevance of the blood and urine levels of mercury that are observed after placement or removal of amalgams, and chewing on amalgam surfaces. In addition, the distribution of mercury into body tissues is highly variable and there appears to be little correlation between levels in urine, blood or hair, and toxic effects.

Acute and chronic toxicity has been reported from exposure to organic and inorganic mercury. These effects of mercury are well documented.

Although cases of allergy to mercury have been reported in the literature, the prevalence of mercury allergy is estimated to be less than 1 percent.

228

In patients presenting a history and/or clinical symptoms of mercury allergy, patch testing may be indicated to confirm the allergy. Because of the infrequency of reports of mercury allergy, it is not recommended that patients be tested routinely for sensitivity. When patch testing is indicated, it is recommended that the patient be referred to a professional trained in the administration and interpretation of the tests.

Information on the effects of measurable blood levels of mercury on the fetus during pregnancy is limited. It is difficult to evaluate the information available because of individual variations in blood levels and the possible association of blood levels with environmental factors such as smoking and ingestion of alcohol and other dietary factors. Additional studies are required before estimates of effect can be made.

Studies in the literature suggest that mercury may affect the formation of T-lymphocytes and imply that an effect on the immune system may be related to diseases of immunologic origin. However, contact allergy, which is T-cell mediated, is the only manifestation that has been documented. The use of T-lymphocytes for diagnosis of allergic conditions should be considered as an experimental procedure. There is a potential for research in this area to estimate whether effects of mercury on T-cells may be a means of early detection of subclinical manifestations of toxicity.

It has been suggested that corrosion of dental amalgam may result in the release of mercury in the oral cavity. This is not considered to be a problem to patients except those who may be hypersensitive to mercury. An additional concern has been expressed that the galvanic current which is produced when dissimilar metals are in direct contact may have an adverse effect on patients. Galvanic current production has been known for over 100 years, and has been the subject of several reports in the literature. However, these reports demonstrate no adverse effect to oral tissues or to the general health of the patient.

On the basis of the information presented in this workshop, there is no documented evidence for recommending the discontinuation of the use of dental amalgams as a restorative material in dentistry. Additionally, the removal of dental amalgam can only be recommended in those patients who have a true hypersensitivity to mercury or other constituents.

COMPOSITE RESTORATIVE MATERIALS

Composite resins may be used effectively in many applications in anterior teeth where the physical properties make it a viable replacement for other materials. However, its use as a restorative material in posterior teeth is currently unacceptable due to problems with excessive wear, other properties and difficulty with placement. It is estimated that the use of composite resins as a posterior restorative material may eventually replace amalgam restorations.

RECOMMENDATIONS FOR FUTURE RESEARCH
OR CLINICAL IMPLEMENTATION

FUTURE RESEARCH

Diagnostic and analytical procedures should be investigated for documenting exposure to metals in alloys.

An evaluation should be made of nickel salts or other nickel compounds which may be formed during the fabrication and use of base-metal alloys.

Investigate the role of nickel, beryllium and chromium as potential carcinogens in dental laboratory technicians.

An assessment should be made of mercury loss from chewing on dental amalgams of different alloy compositions.

Studies should be initiated to determine whether methyl mercury can be formed in vivo.

Epidemiologic studies should be initiated to assess the prevalence of mercury allergy in the United States population.

Biological sampling procedures should be investigated to determine a reliable means of estimating body burden of mercury.

Studies should be initiated to accurately assess blood levels of mercury which may result from dental amalgam.

Research should be initiated to determine whether the effects of mercury on T-lymphocytes may be a means of early detection of sub-clinical manifestations of mercury toxicity.

Studies should be initiated to develop more definitive tests for determining the hypersensitivity to metals used in dentistry.

Studies should examine the potential that thyroid gland enlargement may be an early predictor of mercury intoxication.

Studies are encouraged to determine whether a relationship exists between maternal exposure to mercury and teratogenesis.

The effects of conditions which accelerate corrosion of dental materials on the release of metal ions should be studied in more detail.

The composition of corrosion products should be identified as well as the effect they may have on oral tissues.

Continued research is recommended on the development of alternative restorative materials.

CLINICAL IMPLEMENTATION
There is a need by dentists and physicians to recognize nickel as a common allergen.

Manufacturers, laboratories and dentists should be encouraged to identify alloys used in the fabrication of prosthetic devices in terms of contents which may affect a patient's health (nickel, chromium, cobalt, etc.).

Dentists and administrators of dental laboratories should be encouraged to inform employees who work as technicians regarding the need to avoid inhalation exposure to dusts from alloys.

Practitioners are encouraged to document in patient records content of alloys used in restorative materials.

Health histories should include documentation of individuals sensitive to metals.

Patch testing for sensitivity to metals is the responsibility of professionals trained in the administration and interpretation of the tests.

Practitioners are encouraged to become familiar with the symptoms of metal exposure.

Practitioners are encouraged to report case histories of adverse reactions to or effects from biomaterials to the American Dental Association.

And finally, we would like to share a few quotations from the July 30, 1984 issue of "ADA News", the biweekly issue of the newsletter of the American Dental Association.

The title of the article: Workshop Reaffirms Dental Amalgam Safety

"While reaffirming dental amalgam as a safe and effective restorative material for the majority of Americans, the workshop recommended it may be necessary to consider the removal of amalgam restorations in the small segment of the population that may be hypersensitive to mercury and that exhibits clinical symptoms of a reaction to mercury. This group was estimated to be less than 1 percent of the population."

"The conclusions presented by the planning committee were not intended to represent a consensus of the workshop of about 200 participants, but were based on the information presented. An exception to the general thrust of the conference was made by Dr. Hal Huggins of Colorado Springs, CO."

"Dentists individually and through local, national, and international groups are continuously researching and evaluating the potential hazard of mercury, to both dental patients and dental office personnel."

"There is no scientific evidence that dental amalgams are a health hazard for the vast majority of dental patients."

"So far, the only hazard that has been documented is the hypersensitive reaction of some patients to dental amalgam restorations."

Many people read the title words, "Reaffirms Dental Amalgam Safety", breathed a sigh of relief and disregarded the article. Some people look for reasons behind conclusions. One such person is Dr. Victor Penzer. He was so disgusted with the article that he took the time to fire off his opinion to the ADA. It read as follows:

DR. VICTOR PENZER
197 Grant Avenue
Newton, Massachusetts 02159

Telephone (617) 332-1234

August 8, 1984

Editor, A.D.A. News
211 East Chicago Avenue
Chicago, IL 60611

Re: "Workshop reaffirms amalgam safety"
A.D.A. News, July 30, 1984.

Dear Sir:

What possibly could justify the above headline of your article by an anonymous author? Certainly nothing that transpired in the Workshop proceedings. The participants agreed that biocompatibility of amalgam demands further inquiry. They recommended several specific aspects of toxicity for future research. This alone indicated that they could not in good faith reaffirm amalgam safety. The utmost that the defenders of amalgam managed to insert in the concluding statement was that: "sufficient documented evidence to warrant discontinuing use of dental amalgam does not exist". Yet, with the knowledge of mercury toxicity beyond any dispute, with the modern instrumentation that measures and documents intraoral mercury vapor levels way above the industrial safety limits in the mouths filled with amalgam, and with the clinical and epidemiological reports of amalgam morbidity, we dentists who are determined to heed The Oath of Hippocrates have no other choice but to demand that sufficient documented evidence of safety be provided as a condition for the continuing use of amalgam in humans.

Sincerely,
Dr. Victor Penzer (MD, DDS)

INDEX

M

Magnesium, 94
Manganese, 60, 92
Mercury in blood, 137
Mercury in dental offices, 157, 158, 160, 162, 164
Mercury leaching out, 11, 136, 146
Mercury sources, 100-102
Mercury vapor, 9, 27, 57, 59, 135, 136, 188, 199, 192
Methyl mercury, 29, 30, 31, 69, 127, 137, 149, 151, 155, 194
Mononucleosis, 41, 126
Multiple sclerosis, 18, 29, 30, 37, 38, 148, 153
Multiple Sclerosis Society, 155
Murphy, Doty, 76

N

National Association of Dental Surgeons, 12
Neurological, 32, 37, 139
NIDR, 18-22, 67
Nickel crowns, 41, 106, 127
No touch techniques, 11, 34
Nutrition, Chapter V

O

OSHA, 27, 28, 47

P

Patch test, 53, 198
Periodontal disease, 29, 134, 152
Pernicious anemia, 175, 177
Pinto, Olympio, 8, 13, 14, 16, 44, 63, 68, 171-185, 187
Pleva, Jaro, 30, 85, 141, 193
Pork, 63
Potassium, 61, 95
Protamine zinc insulin, 72, 80
Psychological testing, 75

Q

Questionnaire, 72, back cover

R

Red blood cells, 151, 155
Reese, Joyce, 18, 186

Retention toxicity, 67, 201
Retina, 211
Risk of amalgam, 9
Root canal fillings, 108, 126, 155

S

Schoonover, 68
Scrap amalgam, 34
Sequential amalgam removal, 35, 67-72, 78
Serum proteins, 57-60, 88-90
Sharma, 32
Sodium, 96
Stock, Alfred, 13, 32, 65, 135, 139, 166, 200
Streptococcus muntans, 30, 69, 216
Svare, C., 28, 135
Suicide, 38, 122
Supplementation, 78-81, 114

T

Temperature, body, 76, 197
Thermography, 211, 212
Total protein/globulin ratio, 203
Trachktenberg, 32
Treatment, Chapter 8
Triglycerides, 56, 83, 87
Twenty-one day cycle, 74

U

Universal reactor, 42, 49, 129
Urination, 50
Urine testing, 52, 65-67, 161, 209

V

Vision, 76-77
Vitamin B-12, 204
Vitamin C, 54, 56, 85

W

West, 35
White blood cells, 42, 43, 57, 62, 66, 188, 206

Z

Zinc, 61, 94